Endorser

Beni's new book, *Healthy and Free,* has given me back the hope I needed to bring change into my busy lifestyle. Her journey leaves the reader no excuses for change not to occur. Beni is the perfect motivator. Not only has she done most of the work for us in research, but she has also become a trustworthy example of lifestyle change, proving that change can happen.

TRISHA FROST
Co-author of *Unbound: Breaking Free of Life's Entanglements*
Co-Founder of Shiloh Place Ministries

Two things caused us to shout a big AMEN to Beni Johnson's new book *Healthy and Free.* The first is this: As you get older, you definitely need to pay more attention to exercise, health and nutrition…if you want to maintain your quality of life. And so we really needed to hear her encouragement. Second, because much of our ministry involves prayer for healing, we are amazed at how people are hoping that God will miraculously offset all of their bad habits and wrong choices regarding health and disease issues. A big part of folks staying healthy and keeping their healing is to stop doing the things that made them ill in the first place. To continue abusing our bodies with wrong eating habits, poor sleeping patterns, inactivity, and indifference toward being fit is a downward spiral.

In *Healthy and Free,* Beni will walk you through life-saving essentials working with exercise and nutrition to keep you healthy, and to seriously "up" your quality of life.

Do what she says. Your body and your family will thank you.

JOHN and CAROL ARNOTT
Catch the Fire, Toronto

Hats off to Beni Johnson and her latest book *Healthy and Free!* This is a necessary book for…well, for everyone! We are so happy that Beni is restoring the biblical truths regarding God's will for your body and how you can work with God to ensure divine health.

Healthy and Free is filled with practical steps that will work for any person who wants to get their body functioning at optimal levels. We loved reading it and are already putting its simple advice into practice. People everywhere will be happier, healthier, and freer because Beni Johnson has championed God's original design for healthy living. Thank you, Beni, for giving us this fantastic guide to a fuller life.

WESLEY and STACEY CAMPBELL
www.beahero.org

I have so enjoyed reading Beni Johnson's new book, *Healthy and Free*. I personally have been encouraged, convicted, awakened, and inspired to actually walk out these pages. The Church is in desperate need of a health overhaul. I believe this book is the word of The Lord "for such a time as this." It has personally encouraged me to take care of my body, the tabernacle where Holy Spirit dwells. I wish it was as simple as Beni praying for me and imparting health, muscle mass, and a desire to exercise—but it doesn't work like that. I have to actually "do the stuff." As I read her book, I realized that our health journey doesn't have to be hard. I can do this. We can do this. Let's learn from someone who listened to the Lord and took her health seriously and then wrote it down so we could learn from it and run with it. Read this book. Let's sign up for an incredible journey of being *Healthy and Free*.

JULIE MEYER
Healing Rooms House of Prayer of Santa Maria, California

The one thing better than divine healing is divine health. This kind of health requires most of us to make lifestyle changes in our thought life, behavior, and diet—and even in our walk with the Lord. I have watched Beni pursue this in her devotion to Christ. He is the one who asked her to discover His wisdom for health so that she would be around for "the long haul." This journey is her offering to the Lord.

Healthy and Free is simple, profound, and very encouraging, as she has found keys that are very doable for the average person. As an observer and participant, I can say with certainty that God is doing wonders through her to make this life one of joy, discovery, and blessing. Welcome to the journey!

BILL JOHNSON
Bethel Church, Redding, California

Healthy and Free will save your life! Beni Johnson has written an amazing book that will revolutionize the way you feel, look, and live if you apply the rich truths in *Healthy and Free*. This book may be the most important book for this generation to live an abundant life because it will help them fulfill their God-given destiny and finish well by living a long and healthy life.

DR. CHÉ AHN
Founding Pastor, HRock Church, Pasadena, California
President, Harvest International Ministry

Beni Johnson is an amazing woman who has dedicated her life to walking in health as well as the ministry of healing. She is a wealth of information on the spiritual and natural aspects of how to take care of your body. My wife, DeAnne, loves to talk with Beni and hear her insight about health, exercise, nutrition, and psychological health related to spiritual principles. I highly recommend to you *Healthy and Free*, a book that is easy and enjoyable to read, one that I believe could cause a lot of healing to come to the church.

RANDY CLARK
Founder and President, Global Awakening
Author of *There Is More!* and
Essential Guide to the Power of the Holy Spirit

Healthy & Free

DESTINY IMAGE BOOKS BY BENI JOHNSON

The Happy Intercessor

The Joy of Intercession

The Joy of Intercession Curriculum DVD

The Joy of Intercession Participant's Guide

Healthy & Free

A JOURNEY TO WELLNESS FOR YOUR BODY, SOUL, AND SPIRIT

Beni Johnson

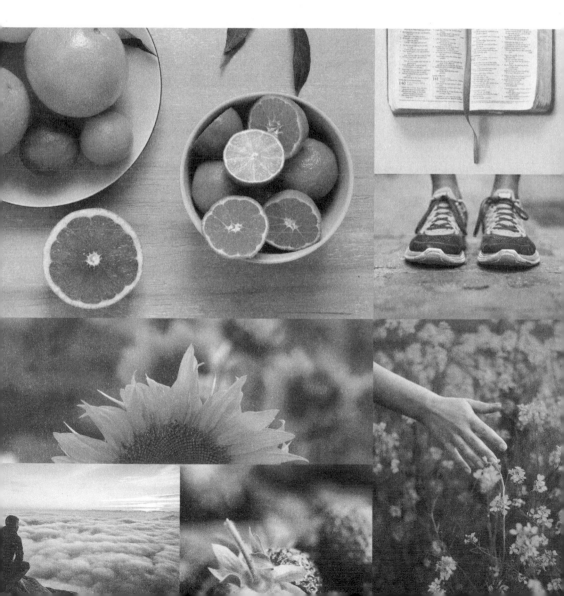

The information contained in this book is the opinion of the author and is for educational purposes only. It is not intended to prescribe, treat, prevent, or diagnose any disease or condition. The Food and Drug Administration has not evaluated many of the therapeutic suggestions and statements offered by the author, particularly not those about essential oils.

DESTINY IMAGE® PUBLISHERS, INC.

P.O. Box 310, Shippensburg, PA 17257-0310

"Promoting Inspired Lives."

This book and all other Destiny Image and Destiny Image Fiction books are available at Christian bookstores and distributors worldwide.

Cover design by Bethel Media

For more information on foreign distributors, call 717-532-3040.

Reach us on the Internet: www.destinyimage.com.

ISBN 13 TP: 978-0-7684-1033-4

For Worldwide Distribution, Printed in the U.S.A.

2 3 4 5 6 7 8 / 19 18 17 16 15

Dedication

Dedicated to those who have stepped into hope and found that nurturing their body, soul, and spirit is a divine assignment. And, seeing the results and pushing through even in the hard times is worth every moment. You all are an inspiration.

Special thanks to Christina Manning Lebek. Your editing was brilliant. We will never forget the word astounding. To Larry Sparks who was so encouraging in this project. To my amazing husband who listened and is willing to try new things. And, to Rihanna Teixeira, your help with research and writing made this project fun. Thanks for the hours you spent. I couldn't have asked for a better person for the job.

Contents

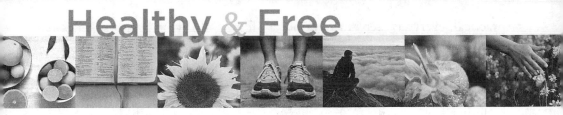

Foreword

Living a healthy lifestyle is a journey. It's not a quick fix. It's not a New Year's resolution. It's not even getting swept up in the latest diet fad. Too many people give up on their health program or diet so quickly, not because the life change is impossible, but because of a wrong perspective; they don't see it as a journey. Every step toward living Healthy and Free should be taken with intentional discipline, clear vision, and a little bit of grace.

When I first heard that Beni Johnson was releasing a book about her personal journey to wellness in body, soul, and spirit, I couldn't have been more excited. What thrills me the most is the impact that Beni's personal journey will have on a whole new generation of believers who seek to live in harmony with God in body, mind, and spirit. Through Bethel Church, she has been given a voice of global influence—what an amazing decision to use her influence to help people around the world, particularly the church, to start walking in divine health—body, soul, and spirit.

It's also refreshing to see a key leader of a movement known for its incredible healings and miracles encourage readers to take the practical, everyday steps to walk out a lifestyle of divine health so that their bodies can be protected from sickness. While many Kingdom leaders have delivered outstanding resources on releasing divine healing—how to administer the miracle-working power of God to those suffering from sickness—Beni has written a reader-friendly blueprint for how to walk in divine health.

As Christians, we have been called to live with excellence. Health and wellness are not just good ideas—they were God's ideas from the beginning. Written with genuine compassion and love, Beni transparently shares her own journey to healthy living. She explains how important it is to find your "why"—your personal motivator for beginning your own journey to health. Her words are also seasoned with much grace. For those who have tried and failed, Beni's approach is warm, practical and user-friendly: There is grace for you to get back up and keep moving forward!

Healthy and Free is not your typical "health book." It's not simply Beni's personal story and it's not a compilation of assorted tips on how to live healthy; it's both. Beni not only shares her story; she shares her story from her own struggles and resulting transformation. Yet, Beni will be the first to say that she doesn't have all the answers and is still learning and experiencing God's health principles herself each and every day. Everything that she shares with you, the reader, she has either done, is currently doing, and has researched. Using an engaging blend of Scripture, relevant health information, exercise recommendations, recipes, and practical tips to get started, Beni delivers a unique book that is certainly a first of its kind.

Wherever you are on your personal health journey, this book will remind you of your personal why, release God's amazing grace over areas you might have let slide, and encourage you with the strength to keep moving forward. I recommend this book because I highly recommend the author. Beni paints an excellent picture that truly reveals God's heart for us when it comes to our physical, spiritual, and mental health. You truly cannot have one without the other, and this book introduces you to health in all three areas: body, soul, and spirit.

I encourage you to receive the invitation that the Holy Spirit is extending through this book. He alone will lead you to success on this journey. In my own journey, I tried dozens of different diets and "miracle cures" in the hope of finding an answer. After two years of unsuccessfully searching for the cure-all, I discovered that God has given us the answers all along. I learned that physical health is a spiritual responsibility. In *Healthy and Free,* you will find the tools that you need to help uncover the knowledge and wisdom that God has given us in His Word to successfully live healthy and full lives.

JORDAN RUBIN
New York Times best-selling author, *The Maker's Diet*

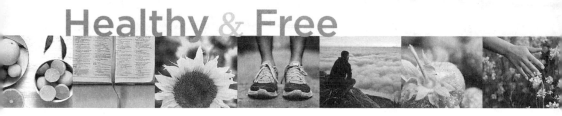

Introduction

In all your ways acknowledge Him,
and He shall direct your paths.
—Proverbs 3:6, NKJV

This book is about my story. It has been a journey full of experiment-ing, soul-searching, and pressing into God. For me, these past years have really been a time of discovery. I've taken an inventory of my thoughts, mindsets, and belief systems and changed many of them so that I can live a full and healthy life in my body, soul, and spirit. New and exciting information regarding health and wellness are discovered on a daily basis as ideas, research and revelations are explored world-wide and I continue to learn so much along the way. Though I never have and never will claim to be a health expert, especially since this subject is ever-changing and growing, this book is about the journey I have taken toward health with the Lord. I want to invite you into my story and to encourage you in your own. My heart is to bring light to those who are searching and to create awareness about how we can take ownership of our lives and our health in all aspects of our body, soul, and spirit. If we lean into God, He will direct our paths.

> *Good friend, don't forget all I've taught you;*
> *take to heart my commands.*
> *They'll help you live a long, long time,*
> *a long life lived full and well.*
> *Don't lose your grip on Love and Loyalty.*
> *Tie them around your neck; carve their initials on your heart.*
> *Earn a reputation for living well*
> *in God's eyes and the eyes of the people.*
> *Trust God from the bottom of your heart;*
> *don't try to figure out everything on your own.*
> *Listen for God's voice in everything you do, everywhere you go;*
> *he's the one who will keep you on track.*
> *Don't assume that you know it all.*
> *Run to God! Run from evil!*
> *Your body will glow with health,*
> *your very bones will vibrate with life!*
> *Honor God with everything you own;*
> *give him the first and the best* (Prov. 3:1–9, MSG).

To your health!

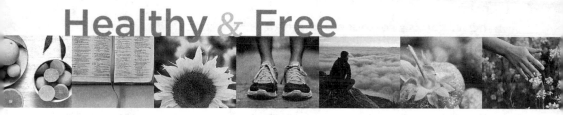

Chapter 1

The Journey

The journey is the treasure.
—LLOYD ALEXANDER

It was the summer of 2004. My husband Bill and I had just moved into our home in west Redding, California. We had spent the past 18 years of our lives pouring ourselves into the renewal movement that had taken place in our church. Life was busy, fast-paced, challenging, and exciting at the same time. A lot of nights, our church meetings would last until well past midnight. Then, we would take our tired bodies to a favorite restaurant and eat big meals just before heading home to go to bed. Although I wasn't aware of it at the time, I was sacrificing my physical health for the sake of my spiritual health, rather than taking into consideration the importance of both.

It all caught up with me one day in my doctor's office. Not only was I 28 pounds overweight, but I had also developed hypertension, which had run in my family. A fancy word for high blood pressure, hypertension is a condition that causes the arteries to elevate your blood pressure—creating more work and tension for your heart.

As I thought about the road ahead of me, I looked back and remembered when I used to lead a fairly healthy life. In the late '80s and early '90s, my husband and I were pastoring a small church in the mountains of Northern California. Bill and I decided to change our diet, based on the nutritional knowledge that we had at the time, and we began to eat healthier. We involved our kids in our choices and began taking our two boys, who were old enough, to the gym to work out with us. Fitness and health became a lifestyle, one that we enjoyed immensely. Finally, I had come to a place where I was comfortable and confident in my body. So, what changed?

As I said, our lives had become very busy as the renewal movement progressed and little by little I had stopped taking care of myself. I was no longer exercising because I felt that I didn't have the time, and I sacrificed life-giving foods for convenience. Before I knew it, I had gone from a size 5–6 to a size 12–13, in just a few years. Now, here I was in my doctor's office facing the fact that my lack of self-care had resulted in weight gain and hypertension.

I decided that I didn't want to resort to taking medications. I had witnessed the struggles of a family member who had taken that path and I knew that there were alternative ways to treat hypertension. I began to do my own research and I found that there is an abundance of health-related information out there. I knew that this was going to require me to lean into the Lord for His guidance and wisdom.

A few months had passed, and though I had made some changes in my lifestyle, they were not the right ones. One morning, as I began to go about my day, I heard the Lord say to me while I was in the kitchen, "I want you to get into shape because I need you around for the long haul." I knew then that a drastic change needed to be made in my life. I couldn't do enough to just get by; I needed to make changes that would fully sustain me. This became my reason "why."

Finding Your "Why"

I teach a health and wellness class at the church where my husband and I pastor. During one of the classes, a man stood up and shared his story about his journey toward wellness. In 2006, he was 130 lbs overweight. Within the space of a week, his girlfriend of two years broke up with him and his doctor told him that he was a high-risk candidate for diabetes. This was a turning point, forcing him to take an honest look at his life. In those two cataclysmic moments of his life he decided that he didn't want to be overweight anymore. Not now, and not again. He had to align his reason for wanting to get healthy with what he felt God had called him to do with his life. This became his "why." I loved the concept of having a "why" and adopted this way of thinking for myself.

When people approach me searching for advice on the best way to get started on a healthy lifestyle, they expect me to tell them to cut out all sugar from their diet or to eat their weight in fruit and vegetables. While I do advise eliminating sugar and eating a fair amount of green, leafy vegetables, my first piece of advice is to find the reason "why" they are embarking on this journey.

Ask yourself this—Why do you want to get healthy? Why do you want to be strong? Why do you want to lose weight? I think it's important to know why you are doing what you are doing. When the Lord spoke to me that morning, years ago in my kitchen, what He said became my "why." I want to become healthy because I want to be around for the long haul. More times than I can count, remembering my "why" has given me the strength to push forward on my journey. It's much easier to say no to a milkshake, a burger with a large side of fries and my old beloved friend, the donut, because I know that they won't help me stay true to my "why."

I remember one particular morning when I was reluctantly driving to the gym and everything inside of me wanted to turn my car around, go home and plop down in front of my television. To be honest, if I hadn't had a meeting with my trainer that day; I don't think I would have made it to the gym. But, on my drive there I was reminded of my "why." I thought back to the day in my kitchen, and the way it felt when God told me so very clearly that He wanted me around for the long haul. Remembering His words and the way that they had resonated with my spirit, I made the decision to give my all at the gym that day. It ended up being one of my best workouts ever. I believe that my willingness to persevere pleased the heart of God and in turn He partnered with my strength.

As you begin your own journey, I can't stress enough the importance of finding your "why." I promise you that it will help get you through many challenges along the way. Maybe you want to become healthier because you'd like to be able to walk your daughter down the aisle at her wedding, or maybe you want your children to experience what it's like to have a parent who can play with them. Everyone has a different "why." Don't wait until you are sick and the doctor has to give you your "why." Find your "why" with God, now.

What's Next?

At times, health and wellness can be overwhelming topics to research because there are so many conflicting ideas out there. I think this is one of the main reasons why many people procrastinate pursuing a healthy lifestyle. I want to encourage you to take baby steps along the way. Remember, this is a journey and not a race. One healthy meal won't solve all your problems, just like one unhealthy meal won't make you fat. It's a day-by-day, moment-by-moment, walk with the Holy Spirit. One thing that I learned in the very beginning of this journey was that if I was willing to partner with the Holy Spirit and lean on Him—He would be faithful to give me the instruction and counsel that I needed. After all, He is called the Great Counselor.

A friend of mine told me what has become one of my favorite stories regarding God's faithful guidance in this area. He had felt from the Lord that he needed to be tested for adrenal fatigue. This condition can occur when prolonged stress is placed on the adrenal glands, resulting in illness, exhaustion, and depression. In some serious cases a person can take two to three hours just to get out of bed in the morning, due to extreme exhaustion.[1] Unfortunately, although many people experience this, adrenal fatigue has not yet been recognized as a medical condition, which means that many doctors will not test for it. However, my friend knew that he had heard from the Holy Spirit, so he persisted. Eventually his doctor ran the tests and sure enough, he had adrenal fatigue.

I am sure that many of you reading this are interested in learning more about adrenal fatigue, which I will talk about more in a later chapter. My point in telling you this story is to encourage you that the Great Physician will lead and guide you as you pursue greater health. There have been times without number when I have heard the Holy Spirit speak to me about certain aspects of my health, only to have my naturopath later confirm what God said to me.

This is just another way that I experience God's love. I remember when I was a teenager, my heart was sold out to Jesus and I would spend time soaking in His Presence, asking Him about anything and everything. I loved hearing Him respond. Sometimes, I would even go into my closet and ask Jesus what He thought I should wear, which, to a teenage girl, is a very important question to ask! I know that may sound extreme to some, but it was such a vital and beautiful part of my growth in the Lord. As I got older, I discovered that God is passionate about me and cares about my health in every area of life.

Now, as an adult, very little has changed. Toward the beginning of my journey, I remember walking into my kitchen and saying out loud, "Where do I start, God?" Immediately, He responded, saying, "Get off sugar." I loved sugar—good old refined white sugar. At that time it could have been classified as one of my main food groups. Being real, I must tell you that there was a time in my life when you'd regularly find me sitting down on the couch with a pound of chocolate tucked tightly into my arms. I would blissfully eat the entire thing, only to be sick and ashamed of myself later—that's the cycle of addiction. I knew that

I needed help and that God would have to intervene in order for me to have the strength to give up sugar.

I began the process of eliminating it from my diet. It was a long two months filled with headaches, body aches, cravings, and cleansing my body before I began to feel the difference. After the initial withdrawals, I felt as though I had just jumped a huge hurdle. Not only had I successfully conquered one of my greatest weaknesses, I felt good physically, as if my body was cleaner and lighter. How in the world did I break this addiction? Well, I took baby steps. First, I found a great supplement (a subject that I will address later in this book). Then, I started adding more vegetables to my diet, especially dark greens because they have components that may help reduce sugar cravings. Also, I began exploring alternatives to refined sugar, such as pure maple syrup, local raw honey, and Stevia. In my experience, the very best way to beat sugar cravings is to drink fresh, organic green juices. Even now, if my sweet tooth is tempting me with my favorite dark chocolate, I will get my juicer out and make myself a tall glass of one of those amazing, dark green juices. I should note that from time to time I do allow myself to eat dark chocolate. It has many great health benefits, and I go by the rule, "The darker the better!"

Changing Your Mind

Next to finding your "why," the single most important thing to becoming healthy is the willingness to change your mind. Many people go into this thinking that at some point, when they reach their goal weight or can fit back into their skinny jeans, they will be able to go back to eating their favorite fried foods or sugary desserts. I am not saying that you will never be able to have the freedom to enjoy those foods again on occasion, but what I am saying is that being healthy is a lifestyle. In contrast, fad diets have a sneaky way of luring people in by promising them fast results rather than long-term change.

I, too, was once a victim of the fad-diet industry. I would start off my new diet strong, but within a few weeks or even just days, I knew that I wouldn't be able to maintain that sort of lifestyle. I would go off my diet, and we all know what happens next—a little thing called out-of-control eating. My experience was like many others'—diets don't work. They were a beginning, but I had to get to the point where I made the decision to change my mind and think about my health differently. This was the moment when I said, "I'm never going back." You see, it had to be a life-style change. If I hadn't listened to God that morning, who knows where I would be.

Grace

Admittedly, I am a stubborn person when it comes to certain things, and my health has become one of those areas. I plan on living for a very long time and I am willing to fight for that. However, this journey is not a walk in the park, and it is certainly not for the faint of heart. Revamping your life and your habits comes with various hurdles that you may need to clear. There will be times when your family and your friends will want you to indulge in excessive meals filled with foods that you know will hurt your body, and you will be faced with a decision. Don't be surprised if you get funny looks or are even teased when you first start making new choices.

At the same time, I never want to be one of those people who lives with such rigid rules that others want to pull away from me, so I allow myself some grace. My husband and I travel quite a bit and we often find ourselves in situations where our meals are prepared for us. In my day-to-day life, I will not budge when it comes to my health, but in these unique situations, when someone has prepared a meal for us, I step into grace. Once, when we were doing a conference in the South, our hosts had an outstanding chef prepare our dinner for us. Southern cooking contains some very delicious dishes, but, being honest, a lot of them are really unhealthy. Sure enough, when we sat down to eat, everything was cooked in fat and smothered in gravy, but I was not about to refuse this dear man's food because I knew that he had worked so hard to bless and please us. For that reason, I stepped into grace and ate a very small portion. (As you might expect, the food tasted amazing.)

So there will be some sacrifices that you need to make, but there will also be times, like my southern experience, where you will have to trust the Lord and indulge a bit. As you step into giving yourself grace, know that He will help keep you on the right path. This is another reason why partnering with God is so vital to your journey. Don't be afraid to ask Him questions and seek His insight just as I did when I walked into my kitchen overwhelmed and confused about where to start. If you let this be a Christ-centered adventure, then I believe that He will give you the supernatural grace to walk it out and see it through. God wants to see us succeed in our desire to be healthy!

Season for Supernatural Grace

When I do any teaching on this subject, I like to end the class with a prayer because I believe in its power to change our hearts as well as the circumstances around us. Prayer is also the act of making an agreement with the Lord and a declaration that we will see a difference in our lives.

If you want to change the journey that you have been on so far into one of health and freedom, then I invite you to pray this prayer, and as you do, know that I am standing in agreement with you:

> *Father, I thank You for the life that You have given to me, and that You intend for me to walk in divine health. Thank You for Your supernatural grace that is a daily gift. Today, I step into that grace in order to become a healthy, whole person. I receive Your counsel and wisdom to choose life, and to walk out the necessary steps for my health.*
>
> *I declare over myself a divine grace to take every step I need to be whole. In Jesus' name! Amen.*

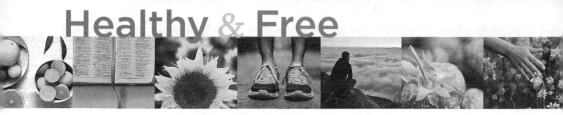
Chapter 2

Soul Health

Happiness dwells in the soul.
—DEMOCRITUS

We use so many different words in reference to the soul that it can become confusing to define it. For example, are "soul" and "spirit" interchangeable? Are "mind" and "soul" the same thing? I found myself thinking about these questions and began to research how they are used in the Bible. An in-depth study of the Greek words for "soul" and "spirit" suggests that they are similar, in fact, almost identical. However, I found this definition, and it helped to clarify the difference for me: The soul is "the essential life of man 'looking earthward' and the spirit is that same principle of life breathed (like wind) into man from God that can look towards and experience God."[1] This suggests that the spirit and the soul have different emphases.

The expression "looking earthward" reminds me of the many positive and neutral experiences, not to mention challenges, that we each face every day. Often, what we think and what we believe can both create situations in our lives as well as determine their outcomes. "Looking earthward" therefore reminds me of expressions such as, "the battle is won or lost in the mind," or "the real war is right between our ears." For the sake of avoiding confusion, I am going to refer to the soul (the part of us that looks earthward) as the mind.

It is important to remember that we are triune beings who consist of a body, a soul (or mind), and a spirit. All three are connected and each one has great importance to God. It can be argued that having a healthy mind is just as important as having a healthy body. In fact, when we have good thoughts about ourselves, it actually causes our whole being to respond in a positive way.

Loving Ourselves

Jesus replied, "You must love the Lord your God with all your heart, all your soul, and all your mind. This is the first and greatest commandment. A second is equally important: 'Love your neighbor as yourself.' The entire law and all the demands of the prophets are based on these two command-ments" (Matt. 22:37-40, NLT).

I love this verse because it so beautifully gives us an important key to living a healthy life. For the second half of the verse to work—for us to love our neighbor as we love ourselves—we first have to love God with our entire being. And loving God isn't something that happens in words but with our actions and our entire lives. Loving God must be something that every fiber of our being can feel. We feel it, we breathe it, and our minds come alive in His love. It's my deep conviction and experience that when you know this kind of love for God you will easily be able to obey the second commandment. The second commandment (note that it is not the second "suggestion") is to love your neighbor as you love yourself. In other words, you have to love yourself first to be able to love others well. There is something about loving God, being loved by Him, loving yourself, and then being able to give that same love to those around you that brings incredible health and life to our lives, and it all starts in our minds.

Giving Yourself Permission

Have you ever seen that YouTube video of the little girl who stands in front of the mirror and shouts everything she loves about herself and her life? She shouts, "I like my hair! I like my haircuts! I can do anything good!"[2] I think many of us adults could learn a valuable lesson from her. We should begin doing the same thing every morning, because we need to start loving ourselves the way God loves us. Do you know that He really does love you, and that knowing this could improve your health? Cognitive neuroscientist and TV host Dr. Caroline Leaf writes, "Being in love creates a positive chemical reaction that causes you to be physically healthier. A lack of love and affirmation can literally make you feel sick."[3] This leads me to wonder if perhaps many of us who are chronically sick would be helped if we learned how to receive God's love and to love ourselves.

Ask yourself these questions: Do I like myself? Do I love myself? If your answer is no, then it is time to give yourself permission to fall in love with yourself. Your entire being is dependent on you to love your mind, body, and spirit. You are worthy of being loved! Be like that girl I referenced in the video! Become like a child and allow yourself to turn those negative thoughts into beautiful words. Doing this will increase your body's innate self-healing ability. A good exercise that I recommend is this: Sit down with a paper and pencil and begin writing down everything that you love about yourself. After you do that, read aloud each thing that you have written about yourself. Some of you may need to really press in and dig deep because you have spent so many years hating yourself. As you begin to say these things out loud, something will begin to change inside of you. You are now giving yourself permission to love you. You are taking charge of your mind and your thoughts.

In her book *Who Switched Off My Brain*, Dr. Leaf states that, "Toxic thoughts are thoughts that trigger negative and anxious emotions, which produce biochemicals, that cause the body stress. They are stored in your mind as well as in the cells in your body."[4] It's time to take these toxic thoughts and replace them with loving ones that will bring us healing.

How Your Mind Affects Your Health

Did you know that your mind can talk you into being fat? Your mind is that powerful! Jon Gabriel, who is a respected pioneer in health and nutrition, believes that in order to really lose weight you have to overcome the lies that you believe about yourself. Gabriel claims that negative and dysfunctional beliefs surrounding obesity and weight loss can activate what he calls FAT programs. These FAT programs are thoughts that literally talk our bodies into resisting change. He writes:

> If you believe that you were meant to be fat, born to be fat, or deserve to be fat, or of you believe that losing weight is difficult or impossible, then your body gets fat or stays fat simply because that's your belief. Weight loss is easy and effortless when you get your body to want to be thin. In order to do this, however, one of the things you have to do is eliminate the dysfunctional beliefs that are getting in your way.[5]

Also, he gives examples of FAT programs that emerge from physical and/or sexual abuse:

> When boundaries are being violated, fat creates a boundary and a shield between you and the abuser. Fat literally puts the abuser farther away. Sometimes in the case of sexual abuse, when you get fat enough, the abuser loses all interest and leaves a person alone.[6]

Because of this, you begin to tell yourself that fat is now your friend and protector—that being fat keeps you safe. Through this, you have talked yourself into obesity as a form of survival.

Stop with me right here and check your thoughts. Ask yourself these questions:

- Do I have thoughts that are keeping me from my goals?

- Are there lies that I believe that are keeping me from a healthy and free life?

- Have I talked myself into believing that I can't reach my goals?

If you said yes to any of those questions, it's time to change the way that you think. First, get out a piece of paper or your journal and begin to ask the Holy Spirit to reveal to you any lies that you may have been believing about your body and your health. Identify those lies and write them down. Next, ask God to show you the truth about yourself. For example, if you are believing the lie that you are unworthy of love because of your weight, repent of that lie and declare the truth that your body shape and size are not what qualifies you to be loved. You are worthy to be loved because Jesus paid the price to qualify you. When you are done, say this prayer:

Father, I see these lies and I now repent from believing these lies about myself. Please forgive me for abusing my mind and my body. I choose to believe what You say about me.

Now, stop and listen to what He is saying to you. Let Him tell you what He is thinking about you. For some, this may be hard and take a little bit of time and that's OK. It is so worth it in the end to be able to walk in freedom apart from those lies. One of the ways that God will partner with you in this journey to health is to give you an entirely new way of relating to yourself.

Changing Your Mind

Don't copy the behavior and customs of this world, but let God transform you into a new person by changing the way you think. Then you will learn to know God's will for you, which is good and pleasing and perfect (Rom. 12:2, NLT).

Did you know that names have a power behind them? I was born and raised in Redding, California. My husband and I had moved away for 17 years, and eventually God brought us back to serve Bethel church. After coming back, I felt that I needed to get reacquainted with my city. I thought that it would help me pray more effectively for this city that I had grown up loving if I knew its history.

I discovered that in the past it had been called Poverty Flats. Once I found this out, I began to notice just how much the events and situations in Redding echoed the economic struggles for which it had always been known. The attitudes of many people were deeply entrenched in a poverty mindset, so much so that when people tried to change the city for the better, there was always a battle. Some did not want the city to change because they were accustomed to the way that it was. Even when a situation is negative, sometimes people will choose not to change. There can be a false sense of safety in sticking with a familiar way of life.

When this historic mentality became clear to us, we began to pray that our city would change its mind. We began with ourselves, and were intentional about changing our thoughts regarding Redding. One of the things that we felt led to pray for was that God would bring a nice department store to the city. There had been a high-end department store that was considering opening a location in Redding, but after doing a study, they discovered that there were too many pizza parlors, a sign of a below-average socio-economic environment, and because of this they did not want to open a store in Redding. We heard the news, but decided to keep praying because we knew that it would help Redding's economy and change the poverty spirit that Redding was accustomed to. I am happy to report that not only do we now have a department store, it is one of the top-performing stores in its chain. We can learn a lot from this story. We decided to change our thoughts regarding the city, and the mentality of our city began to change. We can do the same thing when it comes to our bodies, our health, and our mindsets.

Let's apply this now. Dr. Leaf reports that, on average, we have about 30,000 thoughts a day. When our thoughts are uncontrolled, we actually make ourselves sick. Studies have shown that fear actually causes more than 1400 reactions, both physical and chemical, that activate more than 30 different hormones.[7] Dr. Leaf says, "75%–95% of the illnesses that plague us today are a direct result of our thought life."[8] Wow!

Another important thing to be aware of is the impact it makes when we speak of our conditions with a sense of ownership. How many of us use expressions like *my* weight, *my* eating disorder, *my* high blood pressure, etc.? Your brain listens to those statements, and it believes you. When we own our condition, our brain believes that this is the way we are meant to be, and that the status quo should not change. As you can see, our thoughts have the power and ability to change our lives from the inside out, both for good and bad. If you can relate to any of these ways of thinking, I highly recommend that you study Dr. Caroline Leaf's work. She has some great books as well as an online brain detox.[9]

Repent

The word "repent" in the Greek New Testament simply means, "to turn around."[10] It was once a military term that described a soldier marching in one direction, and then doing an about-face. When this word is used in the spiritual sense, it means to change your mind.[11] Going back to my story about the city of Redding and its former name of Poverty Flats, what I didn't realize was that growing up in that environment had molded me into thinking the same way. I realized this during a time when God began to pour out His physical blessings on our lives in a way that went far beyond my comfort zone. I was lying in bed and I felt the Lord speak to me. He revealed to me that I still had a poverty mindset and it was affecting my response to His desire to bless our family. I immediately repented and began to consciously change my mind. Such a freedom came into my life as a result! I had to make a decision to turn around and think brand-new thoughts about my life and how God wanted me to live it.

If you, too, want to change the direction you are heading and think brand-new, healthy thoughts about yourself, then join me in repenting. Begin anew by starting to make positive declarations over your life.

Declarations

Once you start on the journey to loving yourself, giving yourself permission to change, and doing an "about-face," then you can begin to start making declarations over your life. These are a God-given tool that speak the power of God's Word over ourselves, our lives, relationships, and situations. God created the world and everything we see with a single word. He literally spoke it into existence. So, if we are made in the image of God, and if all authority in Heaven and on earth has been given to us, then our words must be powerful as well. The Bible says, "You will also decree a thing, and it will be established for you; and light will shine on your ways" (Job 22:28, NASB). Declarations come from aligning our thoughts with God's and seeing His will, and then partnering with Him by speaking His truth into existence. A definition of declaration that I love is, "The formal announcement of the beginning of a state or condition."[12] I believe that our words, spoken in faith together with the Holy Spirit, have the power to alter circumstances and change the life course that we are on.

Every morning when we get out of bed, we have a decision to make. We get to choose what kind of day we are going to have. Now I understand that there are days when things take place that are beyond our control. However, I'm talking about normal, day-to-day attitudes that we get to choose each morning. Some days I have woken up and have had to make a conscious choice to choose life. I am a "feeler," and because of that there have been times when it has been hard for me to overcome my emotions and partner with life-giving thoughts. Yet I've learned from experience that whatever emotion I decide to partner with in the morning will most likely be the one that determines the type of day that I am going to have.

What do you want in your life? Happiness? Healthy relationships? You can actually decide to declare those things into existence with holy and godly declarations. Remember that God wants to partner with you, too. He is rooting for you. He is on *your* side. When you begin to unite your declarations with who He says you are, you become a strong and powerful person. Look at these two translations of the same biblical proverb:

> *Death and life are in the power of the tongue* (Prov. 18:21, KJV).

> *Words kill, words give life; they're either poison or fruit—you choose* (Prov. 18:21, MSG).

Wow, what a powerful verse! You and I get to make the crucial choice to speak kindly to ourselves. Unfortunately, many of us have become really good at verbally abusing our bodies, minds, and spirits. It is eye-opening to listen to the harsh and often cruel things that we say to ourselves. If we ask the question, "Would I ever say that out loud to another person?" most of us would answer, "No way!" Yet, we speak to ourselves like this on a daily basis—to this wonderful person that Jesus died for! Thankfully, we can decide to change these negative thought patterns.

In his book *Declarations, Unlocking Your Future,* Steve Backlund says that "declarations are a main building material to frame the 'house' of our destiny."[13] What do you want your life and your future to look like? Start speaking those things to yourself.

To help me with this, one of the things that I have done is to partner with the Holy Spirit, asking Him to reveal to me what His heart is for me. I find it easy to declare the things that He says to me because I know that, above all others, He is on my side.

Laughter

A glad heart makes a cheerful face, but by sorrow of heart the spirit is crushed (Prov. 15:13, ESV).

A cheerful heart brings good healing (Prov. 17:22, NET).

It has been said that laughter is the best medicine, and I have found that to be true in my own life. I experienced this when I was recovering from adrenal fatigue. I had been under so much stress for such a long time that what my body most needed was to relax and laugh! I began making a point to watch hilarious TV shows that crack me up such as *I Love Lucy* and *The Andy Griffith Show*.

A study on laughter found that children laugh around 300 times a day while the average 40-year-old laughs only around four times.[14] We were born to laugh! Anyone who has watched a toddler giggle uncontrollably knows that. Have you ever been in a group of people when a few people start laughing and they cannot stop? Soon the entire group begins laughing, even if they don't know what they are laughing about. That's because God made laughter to be contagious.

I think it is no coincidence that it has many great health benefits. An article titled "Laughter Is the Best Medicine," asserts: "Humor and laughter can strengthen your immune system, boost your energy, diminish pain, and protect you from the damaging effects of stress." Laughter also relaxes the whole body, triggers the release of endorphins, and protects the heart.[15] Amazing!

One of the things that I love about the Holy Spirit is that laughter is so often involved when He manifests in our lives. I believe that God does this for our healing. Do you know that overall feeling of "happy" that you have when you finally stop laughing hysterically? It's a wonderful sensation that helps put everything into perspective. I love how God uses laughter to bring restoration and peace to our bodies and minds.

In addition to declarations, another way to combat lies that you might believe about yourself is to laugh at them. I want to encourage you to do just that. That's right—laugh at them! I know a pastor who strongly believes in this practice, and he will actually put people in a circle, and have each one share with the group a lie that they believe about themselves. As they confess the lie, the whole group begins to laugh. It's a powerful form of ministry because laughter dismantles the lie's power in such a fun way—it reveals the truth, and brings perspective. When I teach on Soul Health, I do the same exercise, and have watched people experience tremendous breakthroughs simply by laughing at the lies that have kept them captive for so long. I highly recommend the book *Let's Just Laugh at That* by Steve Backlund.

I hope that by now you can see just how important the health of your soul is. Since we are triune beings, I cannot stress enough the importance of keeping all aspects of our being healthy and free. When you pay attention to your soul and choose to take steps toward its healing you will find it will be a turning point, not only for your mind, but your body as well.

> *Beloved, I pray that you may prosper in all things and be in health, just as your soul prospers* (3 John 1:2, NKJV).

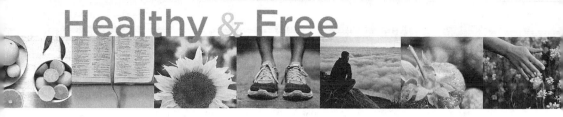
Chapter 3

God's Art

Hope deferred makes the heart sick; but
a dream fulfilled is a tree of life.
—PROVERBS 13:12, NLT

My husband and I travel all over the world speaking in church conferences and gatherings. As you can imagine, we spend a lot of time in
airport terminals. I am a people watcher, and one of my favorite things
to do while waiting at an airport is to observe people. We humans are
brilliant as well as fascinating, and we have so many great qualities.
You can tell a lot about people just by watching their body language
and the way they interact with their family or other travelers.

Another thing that I can't help but notice is that many of us are
sick. Sadly, the same is true for people in the church. It makes me sad
because I feel that those who know Jesus should not only be the hap-
piest, but also the healthiest people on the planet! Now please hear
my heart and know that my intention is not to bring any shame or
guilt to those who are unwell. As I mentioned earlier, my husband

and I love speaking at church conferences, and one of our core beliefs it that if we lay hands on the sick, they can be healed, so I am well aware that there are many reasons why some people are sick and that sickness isn't always self-induced. Regardless, it is important not to feel ashamed, because shame can hold you back, and tempt you to throw in the towel. I want to bring you renewed hope that you can break out of any negative lifestyle or self-defeating pattern in which you feel hopeless and stuck, because then you will have life and joy.

The Great Designer

We are designed by God, who is the greatest artist of all time. We are fashioned with great care and much detail. You are God's best piece of art.

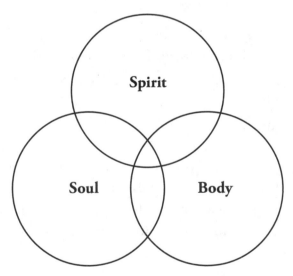

I've always been fascinated with this picture of the body, soul, and spirit. I love the fact that we are made up of all three different elements and they are all connected. In fact, they are beautifully intertwined in a way that leaves no doubt that this was God's creative intention. The word "intertwined" means connected and linked together. In other words, the body, mind, and spirit cannot be separated. This fascinates me, and it leads me to conclude that we are God's greatest creation.

Saving the Best for Last

Many of us are familiar with the story of creation. In six days, God created the heavens and the earth and all things in it. What I find intriguing is that God waited to create His most intricate, complex, and best creation last—us! I'm fairly certain that that's how God works. He saves the best for last.

A similar thing happened in the Gospel of John, when Jesus performed his first miracle:

> *"Now fill your pitchers and take them to the host," Jesus said, and they did. When the host tasted the water that had become wine (he didn't know what had just happened but the servants, of course, knew), he called out the bridegroom, "Everybody I know begins with their finest wines and after the guests have had their fill brings in the cheap stuff. But you've saved the best till now!" This act in Cana of Galilee was the first sign Jesus gave, the first glimpse of his glory* (John 2:8–11, MSG).

In biblical times, the tradition was to serve the best wine first then once everyone had been drinking, they would bring out the less expensive wine. However, Jesus broke with societal norms, as He often loved to do, and created the best tasting wine to be enjoyed last.

The ability to turn water into wine is amazing on its own, but perhaps even more significant is the message contained in this miracle—Jesus reveals His character. More than just a challenge to tradition and human logic, I believe it holds a deeper message. This was a miracle that demonstrated His commitment to excellence and displayed the brilliance of Heaven. People did not expect Him to be able to turn simple water into wine, much less raise the standard by creating the best tasting wine at the end of the party. Yet, that is exactly what He did; He saved the best for last. We recall Jesus' declaration that He only did what He saw His Father doing, and when His Father created the world, He saved the best for last.[1]

Another example of God's unique model of craftsmanship is found in the story of God giving Moses detailed instructions regarding how to build a sanctuary: "Direct them to build a holy sanctuary in My honor so that I can dwell among them. Instruct the people to follow the pattern I am about to show you for the congregation tent and its furnishings" (Exod. 25:8-9, VOICE).

Throughout the chapter, God proceeds to tell Moses all the intricate details and directions regarding how He wanted the sanctuary built. He had Moses pick out just the right wood and fabric, and He even gave exact measurements to go along with His directions. I imagine that the sanctuary was not only breathtaking but also outstanding, because God refused to overlook even the slightest detail. I don't think that He did this because He is a micromanager, but rather to reveal to us who He is as the Master Designer. God loves details. We know this because the Scriptures tell us that not only does God care about us passionately, He even knows the exact number of hairs on our heads![2] When it comes to knowing a person, I don't think that you can get more detailed than that.

Out of all the beauty and wonders that God has created in this world, we are His very best workmanship. The magnificent knowledge and care with which He formed us leaves me speechless. We truly are His best design, His perfect piece of art. In the beginning, God created majestic mountains, vast and incredible seas, rivers that run with power and strength, and skies that hold infinite mysteries, but that was still not enough to satisfy the heart of God. So, He created people. He saved His best for last.

Triune Being

As God was creating the world, He made a very interesting decision. He said, "Let Us [Father, Son, and Holy Spirit] make mankind in Our image, after Our likeness" (Gen. 1:26).

Just as the Father, Son, and the Holy Spirit are a triune God, we are also created as triune beings. We are composed of body, soul, and spirit. The beauty and mystery of the Godhead is that there is no separation between the three. They are different and yet the same. Since we are made in His image, the same is true for us. There is no separation between our bodies, souls, and spirits. We have to see ourselves as this whole being, and appreciate how God made us, without elevating one part over another.

Bill and I both love great artwork and have several pieces exhibited in our home. Whenever we get a new painting, we always know exactly where we want it to be hung in our home. We would never purchase an expensive piece of art only to carelessly drag it to our car, throw it in the backseat, and bring it home to leave it in the garage where it would sit forgotten and collecting dust. Doing that would not only damage the artwork, but it would offend the artist. We want it to be on display for everyone to see! The same is true with God. We are His beautiful artwork made with great design and detail. Every cell, muscle, and organ has been strategically woven together. When we abuse our bodies, we are abusing the very thing that God tenderly and brilliantly crafted: "For you created my inmost being; you knit me together in my mother's womb" (Ps. 139:13, NIV).

God has authored our human development from the very beginning. The Bible says that He fashioned us in our mother's womb. Wow! I'm sure that every young parent can relate to the overwhelming joy and wonder that you felt the first time you saw your baby in an ultrasound. Every few months you would get to witness your baby growing and maturing in the womb. Every day something was developing in the baby. That is God's handiwork. From the first moment of our existence, He has been creating and fashioning us with great excitement and love. We are His great design.

Growing up, science was always one of my favorite subjects. I especially find human anatomy fascinating because of how intricately God puts us together. As I continue to study the human body, learning how tissues, organs, muscles, and nerves work together in harmony, I am continually brought to a place of awe as I think about how great God is.

Science has always brought me closer to God as I find myself offering up thanks to the Great Designer for His ingenuity and amazing plan.

Our Blood

One of my favorite examples of this is the way that He designed our blood, which is made up of white and red blood cells and plasma. Blood is the most commonly tested part of our bodies. Often referred to as the river of life, every cell in our bodies depends on it to meet a variety of needs. It carries away waste as well as provides oxygen and nutrients to every cell in our bodies. White blood cells move throughout the body as a vital part of our immune system, working to protect us from disease, infection, and sickness. By circulating throughout the body, they go directly to the areas where they are needed to fight off infections. The red blood cells carry oxygen throughout the body, and they also carry off carbon dioxide. Amazingly, they have no nucleus and can change shape so that they can squeeze single file through the capillaries.

In short, the intricacy and complexity of our bodies is stunning and the more I discover about them, the deeper I fall in love with our Creator. The detail with which He designed us is not only proof of His existence, but also that He truly is in love with us.

Our Muscles

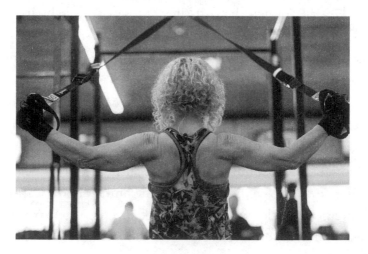

Over the course of my journey into wellness, I rediscovered how much I love working out and keeping my body in excellent shape. I am a bodybuilder and there are few things I love more than getting into the gym and lifting weights. It is extremely important for us to take care of our muscles through exercise, because they have been designed to protect our organs and bones (I will cover more of this topic later in the book). Specifically, I have learned the importance of lifting weights, and to strategically target certain muscle groups during my workouts. One particular day, I was at the gym lifting weights, targeting my back muscles. Our daughter, Leah, was also working out, so I had asked her to take some pictures for me (this is an important thing to do because gauging our progress helps us to stay encouraged in the process). When I arrived home and I looked at the pictures, I was amazed. There were muscles in my back that I didn't even know existed! Once again, I thought about the beauty of how God has designed us, and it gave me a greater incentive to want to take care of this temple that God has specifically given to me to live in. You were each given your own temple that was strategically designed and crafted just for you, and you're the only one who can take care of it. It is easier for Christians to know how to take care of our spirits and minds, but we sometimes forget that it's just as important for us to take care of our bodies. "For no man ever hated his own flesh, but nourishes and carefully protects and cherishes it" (Eph. 5:29).

I pray that as you read this and continue on your journey, the Lord will reveal to you just how perfectly crafted you are—that you are His best work. I pray that you would know the importance of not only keeping your spirit and mind aligned with God, but your body, too. There is a God-ordained balance that He gives us the ability to walk in, and my hope is that you will lean fully into Him to find it so that your body, mind, and spirit are whole in Him.

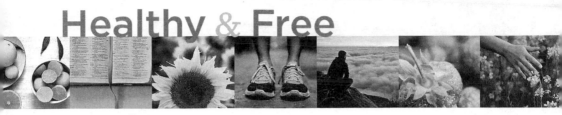

Chapter 4

Tools for Health

I believe that we have been given the tools by God to live successfully. There are simple and practical ways to achieve health and keep your body well and in this section we will explore these tools.

As we go forward, remember that this is not a rulebook you must follow, but rather a guideline inspired by my personal story. These are the foundational tools that I have incorporated into my life, and I hope that, along with the counsel of your healthcare provider, they will help to guide you on your journey.

Let's get started!

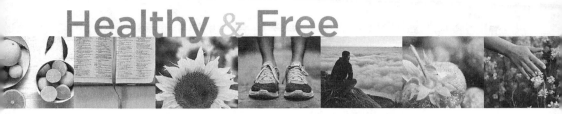

4.1

Hydration

When I am asked what I believe is the most important component of living a healthy life, I always reply, "drinking water." A few years ago, a friend of mine came to me seeking advice on behalf of her mother who had been sick for some time. Her doctor had been unable to find anything wrong with her. It occurred to me to ask her about her water intake. It turned out that not only was she not drinking water, she practically lived on coffee, which only further dehydrates a person! I told her to have her mom drink half of her body weight in ounces of water a day and to give it at least two weeks, and to follow up with me after that. Sure enough, she joyfully told me that not only had her mom's symptoms decreased, they had stopped altogether! The physical problems that we experience often come from a simple lack of hydration.

Water is a vital factor in determining our health for many reasons. Did you know that our bodies are made up of 50 to 75 percent water? Infants' bodies actually have a much higher water content, typically ranging from 75 to 78 percent, which then drops to 65 percent by the time they reach their first year.[1] Body composition and activity level will also affect the percentage of water in your body because fatty tissue contains more water than lean tissue. For example, the body of an average adult male is about 60 percent water while the average female's is 55 percent (because females tend to have more fatty tissue than men do). As a result, those who are overweight will carry more water.[2]

If you feel thirsty, you are already on your way to dehydration, and you will have already lost around 2 to 3 percent of your body's water content. Your mental and physical coordination start to become impaired once your body's hydration drops just 1 percent.[3] Yikes! You can see why staying hydrated is so important.

David Herzog, in his book, *Natural to Supernatural Health*, states that the majority of people are constantly dehydrated. Many don't realize this because they are constantly reaching for a soda or their favorite sugary, caffeinated latte when they feel thirsty, which, unbeknownst to them, only leads to more dehydration. Some will pour themselves a glass of tap water straight from the sink without realizing that they may be drinking chemicals like phosphorous, chlorine, as well as heavy metals and toxins. Dehydration can lead to a variety of sickness, disease, and a slower metabolism.[4] The human body can survive weeks without food, but only three to five days without water before it begins to shut down.

So how much water should we be drinking? A good rule of thumb is to take your body weight, divide it by two, and drink that number in ounces. For example, if you weigh 130 pounds, you should be drinking 65 ounces a day in water. I know that this may seem overwhelming. It did to me! Before I started my journey to health, I, too, did not drink enough water. I didn't like it, and the thought of drinking it bored me. I still remember the day when I purchased a 16.9-ounce bottle of water, and I stared at it thinking that there was no way that I could possibly drink that entire thing in one day! However, being the determined person that I am, I drank the entire bottle. Boy, was it a shock to my system. I became nauseated. However, I knew that hydration would be a key factor in my journey to health, so I continued drinking water.

Over time I began to notice that not only did I love water, but my body loved it as well. I was surprised by how much better I felt when I was hydrated. Today, now that I incorporate an intense workout regimen into my life, I drink about one gallon of water a day. What a change from the woman who was once intimidated by a 16-ounce bottle.

I am intentional about making sure my body is receiving an adequate amount of water. I keep a glass by my bed, so that it's ready for me to drink first thing when I open my eyes. I then make sure to drink another glass of water before I eat breakfast.

Water has been called the Fountain of Youth because without it, nothing is able to survive. Every cell, organ, muscle, and bone thrives on good clean water. In fact, drinking water is one of the best anti-aging regimens. It's the best way to prevent wrinkles, and it's also a lot easier on your bank account than any wrinkle serum you might purchase at a department store!

Water is also our body's main source of energy, sometimes known as the "cash flow" of the body, believed to help the body generate electric and magnetic energy inside each cell. [5] Water helps prevent DNA damage and makes the body's repair mechanisms more efficient. It also increases the efficiency of the immune system in the bone marrow (where the immune system is formed), and assists its effort to fight cancer.[6] Water aids in the digestive process and helps the body convert food into energy.[7]

Water is also the most effective lubricating laxative and helps prevent constipation. It serves as a great pick-me-up. If you experience an afternoon slump, and are in the habit of grabbing a coffee or a sugary soda, instead pour yourself a tall glass of cold water, and allow your body to use its favorite source of energy! Women should know that water also helps decrease premenstrual pain and hot flashes.

These are just a few examples of how water helps to heal and restore your body. To see more reasons to drink more water, I suggest reading *You're not Sick, You're Thirsty*.[8] Before we move on, why not pour yourself a tall glass of clean water and drink up?

Not All Water Is Created Equal

Water advertisements display snow-topped mountains covered in pine trees, parted by glistening rivers which cascade down into peaceful streams. You can almost smell the fresh forests, and hear the water as it rushes down the mountaintop. These images are meant to give you a sense of peace, in order to lead you to believe that the water you are about to drink comes directly from this scenic wonderland. Unfortunately the reality is that it is actually fairly difficult to find pure water today. Even home wells, which were once the most trustworthy water sources for many families, have now become contaminated. The reason for this is that today's agriculture and consumer products are saturated with chemicals. In 1968, the United States hit a milestone when it manufactured its one-millionth chemical. Yes, you read that correctly. As bad as that sounds, it gets worse. As of February 2006, there were 8,369,477 man-made chemicals commercially available for use in our food and beverage products. In a government report, it was found that there are over 2,000 chemicals found in our drinking water alone.[9] I am not going to go into great detail because to do so would be a book in itself, but I would like to discuss a few significant chemicals that we must be educated about.[10]

Chlorine

Bad bacteria love to gather within water, especially water that has been sitting. So, chlorine gets added because it acts as a purifying agent to kill the bacteria. This is a double-edged sword because although we do want the bacteria in our water eliminated, we are now left with a man-made chemical that is not entirely safe to ingest. When combined with organic materials, chlorine forms cancer-promoting trihalomethanes, which may be why studies have suggested a link between chlorine and different kinds of cancers, birth defects, miscarriages, and spina bifida. Chlorinated water also destroys the nutrients that your body needs to thrive such as vitamins A, B, C, E, along with fatty acids. It's also been linked to chronic skin disease, acne, psoriasis, and eczema.[11]

Most of us bathe using tap water, which means that we are putting chlorine directly on our skin and face. Just because you don't directly ingest something by eating or drinking, doesn't mean that it is not still making its way into your body. Our skin is our body's largest organ, and it soaks up everything we apply to it from makeup to body wash to bathing water. I have a filter on my shower, which I've grown accustomed to. Whenever I travel I notice the difference in texture and lack of moisture in my hair and skin. Chlorine also negatively affects your thyroid, which I will go into greater detail later in the thyroid health section of this book.

Fluoride

Fluoride is a toxic chemical found in most of our drinking water. Take a look at your toothpaste and notice the warning labels on the tube. While fluoride does prevent tooth decay, it comes at the price of destroying liver enzymes, adding toxins to your kidney tissues, decreasing fertility rates, and causing negative effects on your pineal gland and melatonin levels (strike a chord with any insomniacs?). It has also been linked to an increased rate of hypothyroidism and to many brain disorders such as Alzheimer's and dementia.[12]

I feel that it is important to note that the reason the government adds these chemicals into our water is in order to protect us from harmful bacteria and other substances, for which I am grateful. However, it is important to be educated regarding your drinking water so that you can decide for yourself what the next healthy step needs to be for you and perhaps for your family.

The Next Step

Like most problems, this one has a variety of possible solutions. Go to any Walmart or kitchen appliance store, and you will find an entire aisle set aside just for water filters ranging in price anywhere from 20 dollars to thousands of dollars. Most of us cannot afford to go out and buy the most deluxe filter due to the expense. However, there are also some affordable options. I have a filtered water machine that my husband and I use for cooking and drinking, but if that is not possible for you, a good start would be a water pitcher system. I have listed a few good filters in the resource section in the back of the book. There are many resources you can find online that can help you find the right water filter for you, which leads me to my next topic. To alkalize or not to alkalize?

The small filtered water machine in our home alkalizes the water. An alkalized water machine divides the acidic water from the alkalized. Our bodies actually need to live in an alkalized state and our pH levels should test out to be between 7.0 and 7.5. I have saliva strips that I use to test my alkalinity levels from time to time.

Even if you aren't able to afford an alkalized water filter, do continue to drink plenty of water. It's more important to be hydrated than to be afraid of what may be in your drinking water and become dehydrated. Thankfully, there are a few ways that you can alkalize your water without a fancy machine. For example, fresh lemons and limes both have alkalizing effects so squeeze a lemon in your next glass of water. An added bonus to adding lemon to your water is that it will do wonders for your digestive system as well.

If you are going to drink bottled water, do your research and make sure that it is actually bottled at the source. I live in Northern California by Mount Shasta, where there is a spring that comes right out of the rock of the mountain. Many families carry big jugs there to fill up with water from this wonderful, clear source.

Water quality can be an overwhelming subject due to the vast amount of information on the topic. In fact, I should note that not everyone agrees about drinking alkalized water. I have a friend who is a naturopath who prefers to drink only spring water. Whether you tend to gravitate toward alkalized or spring water is secondary to the importance of hydration itself. What I hope that you will remember from this chapter is that you must drink, drink, drink!

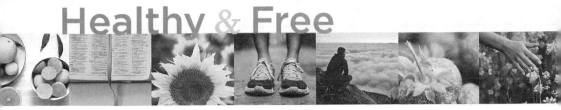

4.2

The Power of Sleep

When I was sleep deprived, I used to dream of a getaway on an exotic island where I could sleep to my heart's content with no disruptions. Many of us at least dream of being able to sleep in without the pressure to get up, make breakfast, take the kids to school, or go to work. Life seems to be so packed full with events and busyness that sleep often takes a backseat. You might be a person who lives a constant, fast-paced lifestyle where there is always somewhere to be or something to do. Perhaps you feel guilty when you start to feel run down and decide to rest because you expect that you should have been able to get by on only a few hours of sleep. Too many of us feel that there are more productive things to do with our time than just sleep.

I used to think that way. I still remember the days when I was a young mom and my life was filled with the constant chatter of children, play dates, diapers, dinners, and the cleaning up of messes. Although my children brought me great joy, I still felt that I needed "alone time" to refuel. Like most parents, I had times when it felt like my life wasn't my own anymore. The only time I could get away by myself was after midnight! So night after night I would stay up until

2:00 A.M. just to be woken up a few hours later. I thought I was giving myself a treat by having alone time, but really I was setting myself up for a perpetual cycle of exhaustion. I now see that sleep would have been a much better treat for my body than a few quiet hours by myself.

We have to change our thinking and allow our bodies to sleep. If you are like I was, I am hoping that this chapter will shed some light on the importance of getting a full night's sleep. Rest, even a power nap, may help improve your health and quality of life dramatically. First, let's talk about the stages of sleep and their importance to our bodies.

Stages of Sleep

Many of us go to bed and wake up the next morning completely unaware of all the work our body just accomplished while we were sleeping. When you give your body a full night's rest, you enable it to go through all four stages of sleep, which is very important for your health. For fun, you can download an app onto your mobile phone called "Sleep Cycle," and it will attempt to monitor your sleep, giving you a better idea of how well you are sleeping.

Stage 1

This is the earliest stage of sleep, and also the easiest one from which to be awakened. During stage 1 sleep, your brain begins to send out slow brain waves called theta waves.[1] If you wake up during this stage of sleep, you may wonder if you have been asleep at all. It's a peaceful state that normally helps clear and calm your mind.[2]

Stage 2

This stage consists of moderately deep sleep, and it's the type that we tend to stay in throughout the night. During this stage, your heart and vascular system slow down and begin to get a well-deserved rest.

Stage 3

This is our deepest sleep, and "it's also called our slow-wave sleep because our brain waves are these slow, high-amplitude waves."[3]

According to the National Sleep Foundation, during this stage it is normal for our blood pressure to drop and our breathing to slow down. This is when our muscles and tissues are repaired. Hormones, primarily the human growth hormone, are produced during this stage. During this phase you will experience the deepest level of sleep, which will help you feel rested and energetic the next day. About 20 percent of your night is spent in stage 3 sleep, which normally occurs in the first half of the night.

Stage 4

Stage 4 is also known as "REM sleep." REM stands for rapid eye movement, and this is when you sometimes experience vivid and imaginative dreams. Your breathing becomes more varied, and your muscle groups become paralyzed which keeps you from acting out your dreams. The first round of REM is typically fairly short and it occurs at the end of the sleep cycle. However, each REM session gets progressively longer throughout the night as your deep sleep (stage three) gets shorter. Dr. Philip Gehrman, assistant professor of psychiatry at the University of Pennsylvania, explains that "most of our deep sleep happens in the first half of the night and most of our REM sleep happens in the second half of the night."[4] During the REM cycle, our bodies and especially our brains are being recharged with much-needed energy.[5] Like deep sleep, only about 20 percent of our night is spent in REM sleep.[6]

Hormones and Sleep

Our bodies recalibrate as we sleep. Our brains, nervous and respiratory systems, and organs are restored. In addition, there are some other great benefits to getting enough sleep. Sleep regulates hormones, such as those that regulate appetite. Leptin and ghrelin are known as the hunger hormones. Leptin is a hormone made by fat cells that decreases your appetite. Ghrelin is a hormone that increases your appetite. Both play a role in your body weight and sleep is the key factor in regulating the two.[7] If they aren't properly regulated, then your body may not be producing enough leptin, which will make you feel hungry when you are not. An increase in ghrelin will also lead to a feeling of hunger. Without a proper balance, weight gain and frustrated weight loss efforts can result.[8]

How Much Sleep

By now I hope I have convinced you that getting a few good *ZZZs* will help you to be healthy. The next question is, "how much sleep?" Well, the ideal amount of sleep is about seven and a half to eight hours, plus an afternoon nap. For many of us, getting that much sleep seems impossible, so my suggestion is to do the very best that you can. I remember speaking to one mom who told me that she hadn't had a good night's sleep in over ten years! It brought me back to the days when I was a young mom, and I used to wonder if I would ever sleep again. I still remember hearing my sweet babies cry in the middle of night, waking from a deep sleep because they needed to be nursed. Sometimes I would grumble as I forced myself out of bed and my husband would have to remind me to calm down. I have always loved to sleep. Many times I made sure that when I put my kids down for their afternoon naps I would take a power nap myself. It's amazing how even just a blissful 20-minute nap seemed to really restore and energize me for the rest of the day.

Sabotaging Your Sleep

I truly believe that when you deprive yourself of sleep you are only setting yourself up to fail physically and sometimes emotionally. I have read many books and heard countless stories of people who spent their lives serving till they came to the end of themselves. Many of them minimized the need for sleep, thinking that it was more important to spend themselves on the needs of others. By putting themselves last, many went into burnout, and some made bad choices. I remember reading a book about a certain minister, who was asked if there was one thing he would have done differently in his life. His answer was, "I should have gotten enough sleep." I believe that sometimes the cause for failure in people's moral lives, ministry, and physical health can be traced back to prolonged sleep deprivation. Otherwise godly people can allow themselves is to become so exhausted that they begin letting their guard down in inappropriate ways. Some individuals I have spoken to who struggle with mental problems have shared that the root of their problems almost always started with a lack of sleep.

The following things have been found to disrupt one's sleep cycle:

- **Stress and anxiety.**

- **Painful physical conditions.**

- **Caffeine:** The average American drinks three cups of coffee a day! Any caffeine increases the stress hormones adrenaline and cortisol that can stay elevated for up to 24 hours.

- **Cigarettes and alcohol:** The nicotine found in cigarettes is a stimulant. Many people use alcohol to help themselves fall asleep. However, alcohol can disrupt your sleep patterns, which causes you to sleep lighter and leads to not feeling refreshed when you awake.

- **Medications:** Many medications have insomnia listed as a side effect.

- **Foods:** Eating high amounts of sugary, processed food may stimulate your brain. That bowl of ice cream, slice of cake, or bag of popcorn before bed stimulates excessive insulin release from the pancreas. I know that if I have any type of carb before I go to bed, I will almost always end up wide awake at 3:00 A.M. and have hot flashes throughout the night.

- **Exercise:** People who exercise three hours before bed raise their levels of stress hormones, which may interfere with their sleep.

- **A bad mattress or pillow:** Having a good pillow is worth its weight in gold. I searched for years to find a pillow that worked for me.

- **A snoring spouse:** As comical as it may sound, this could be a real problem for many couples. There are many solutions out there that may help reduce snoring.

- **Hot flashes or menstrual cramps:** There is nothing worse than being woken up and having to throw off the covers because your body feels like a furnace. Equally difficult is lying in bed with abdominal or back pain. There are solutions that may help with these conditions, which I will cover in another section.

I have a regimen that I follow every night to ensure that I am going to sleep well. As I said earlier, I love to sleep! Because I know my body is restoring itself while I am asleep, I will do whatever is needed to protect my rest! First, I make sure that the last thing I eat is a small portion of protein. This helps aid my body in the sleep process, and it also helps burn fat as I sleep. It might just be a tablespoon of almond butter, some chicken, or some peas, but I make sure I have a bit of protein last thing before bed. On the other hand, I avoid having simple carbs such as bread (even gluten free) or fruit, because they will increase my blood sugar, which could prevent me from getting a good night's rest. I then apply the essential oils cedarwood, lavender, and xlang xlang to my left big toe, and then all over my feet. I do this because our feet are the most porous parts of our body, so they absorb the oils quickly and efficiently. (Read more about essential oils in chapter 6.) I also like to take magnesium because it helps our muscles relax. Sometimes, I take a product called Calm, which is high in magnesium, and also a thyroid supplement called Thyromin by Young Living Oils. On occasion, I use melatonin, especially when I am traveling. However, melatonin is a natural hormone that our bodies should have that helps regulate our sleep/wake cycles. Instead of taking a supplement for it, I recommend sitting directly in the sun during the early morning hours without sunscreen. This helps our bodies absorb vitamin D while regulating our natural melatonin levels.

In summary, I cannot stress enough the importance of good sleep. Sports science researcher Dr. Robert Portman explains the importance of sleep:

> In the daytime, the metabolic processes that control energy, stress, and appetite work best. If we remain awake after nightfall, these metabolic processes become far less efficient. Our normal metabolism gets out of sync, our appetite is turned on so we eat more, we don't convert food to energy, stress levels remain elevated—and we gain weight.[9]

Many people who are dedicated to a healthy diet and exercise but still cannot seem to shake the extra pounds may just need to make sure they are getting enough sleep. Sleep is the foundation for good health because without it, the body simply cannot reap the benefits of a healthy lifestyle. Sleeping will help you mentally and emotionally, too.

Don't be afraid to allow yourself to relax and get a good amount of sleep. Whatever you have on your to-do list will still be there tomorrow when you get up. Only then you'll be well rested and in a better place spiritually, mentally, and physically to accomplish all that you need to get done.

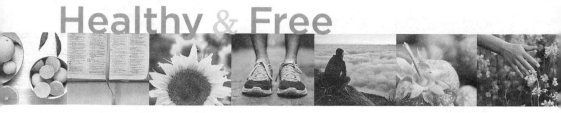

4.3

Get Moving

It is often said, "If exercise were a pill, it would be the most cost-effective drug ever invented."

I assume that everyone has experienced those days when you sit on the couch for hours watching television only to feel stagnant, overtired, and a little foggy-brained. Once we stand up and begin to move around, we start to feel better. This proves that we were not created to be sedentary creatures.

I have always been an active person. While many young girls dreaded PE in elementary school, it was actually my favorite class. I loved being active. I also love nature, and some of my fondest childhood memories are of fun times that I spent outdoors, whether it was playing baseball or tossing a football in my neighbor's yard. I was what you might call a tomboy and I wasn't afraid to play sports with the boys in our neighborhood. I also was known for my love of climbing trees. A perfect afternoon for me would consist of finding a big, tall tree and climbing as high as I could climb.

As children, many of us were naturally active; we would just do the things that we loved. Unfortunately, our physical activity decreases as we mature into adulthood mostly due to the fact that we replaced climbing trees with desk jobs. As a young married couple, Bill and I loved being outdoors and stayed active by playing tennis. We eventually switched to playing racquetball because we liked the fast-paced intensity of it. When we became pastors in Weaverville, California, I joined different sports leagues in town such as volleyball, softball, and even ballet! Ballet is a great workout, but I think my girlfriends and I spent most of the time laughing at each other as we tried to gracefully leap across the room. As I remember it, we more closely resembled a herd of cows than ballerinas, but that is a different story!

After a few years, my husband and I decided to join our local gym. Our two boys would join us every day, and it became a wonderful family activity (Leah, our daughter, was too young to work out at the time). We would go almost every day after school and we worked out about six days a week. That's when I fell in love with lifting weights. I loved the challenge of it along with its detoxing benefits. I found that I am what they call an "easy builder," which means that I can build large muscle mass quickly. I experienced fast results and was amazed at how strong I felt. Now, almost 20 years (and a long break from the gym) later, I find myself loving it again.

Now, do you have to go to a gym to get results? Not at all. I just want to encourage you to move! Whether it's going to the gym, riding a bike, playing sports, or working out in your living room, the sacrifice of exercise is minimal compared to its benefits! I promise that you will not regret it.

Aside from the massive endorphin release that you get from exercise, which makes you feel good, there are many other benefits to living an active lifestyle. A study done by the U.S. Department of Health and Human Services found that the benefits of exercise include:

- An increased chance of living a longer and healthier life.

- Protection from developing heart disease and stroke, and high blood pressure.

- Prevention of certain cancers, including colon and breast cancer, and possibly lung and endometrial cancer.

- Help with the prevention of type 2 diabetes and metabolic syndrome.

- Prevention of osteoporosis.

- Reduced risk of falling and improved cognitive function among older adults.

- Preventing weight gain, promoting weight loss, and help keeping weight off after weight loss.

- Improving heart, lung, and muscle function.

- Improving sleep.

Not only does exercise benefit your physical body, but it also has great benefits for your mind. It has been proven that physical activity can help combat depression and mental fog; it can increase your body image and self-esteem, and it can help relieve stress.[1] Many people who have struggled with drug or alcohol addictions have been able to maintain their freedom because of exercise. In an interesting study done by Vanderbilt University researchers found that when they had asked 12 heavy marijuana users (deemed cannabis-dependent) to run on a treadmill ten times for thirty minutes in a two-week period, their cravings and drug use declined by over 50 percent. They didn't ask them to change anything about their lifestyle other than incorporating physical activity.[2] Regardless of whether or not you may have a drug or alcohol addiction, this study shows the healing power of exercise and its amazing effect on our minds. Just reading that makes me want to get outside and get moving!

I cannot stress enough the value and importance that I place on exercise in my day-to-day life. As I have shared previously in this book, there was a time when I had let myself go for years and neglected taking care of my body through exercise. I always knew that I *should* exercise, but I always found excuses that seemed more important at the time. Excuses come at a price, however. I eventually found myself overweight, feeling sick, and with hypertension. It was remarkable to me how quickly I began to feel better once I made the decision to begin exercising again. This improvement, both mentally and physically, showed me the importance of making sure that I maintain an active lifestyle.

The Importance of Muscles

Why is muscle mass so important? For starters, muscle burns fat. So, if you are trying to lose weight, building your muscle mass will help tremendously. Keep in mind that muscle weighs more than fat, so even if the scale claims that you haven't lost a pound, you will have lost inches. Most of us have seen the picture that compares five pounds of muscle to five pounds of fat. Although both are the same weight, the muscle takes up less room and is lean and firm. Not only is it beneficial for its fat-burning properties, but muscle is your friend especially in the aging process. Around age 40, everyone begins to start losing muscle. The older you get, the more you lose. I am 60 years old as I write this book, which is why building muscle is a top priority for me.

Muscle and Bones

Working out also helps build a strong skeletal system. We may not give a lot of thought to our bones, but they are actually comprised of living tissue that grows stronger with exercise. Regular strength training and other forms of weight-bearing exercise are key to improving the health and strength of our bones by increasing or maintaining (depending on your age) our bone density. Lifting weights has also been shown to reduce the risk of osteoporosis and related fractures.[3] That is why it is so important, especially for women, that they build muscles in order to help with menopause and bone density health. Years ago, I advised my daughter to begin building muscle because it would be the smartest thing she could do for her health. Thankfully, she listened and has gone on to become not just an avid weight lifter but a competitor, too. She is young now, but when she reaches my age she will be far ahead of her peers and will not have to be concerned with her bone density or disintegration of her muscle mass.

Types of Exercise

What types of exercise should we consider, and why?

Cardio

Doing cardiovascular (cardio) exercises should be an important part of your exercise routine. It has many benefits that include promoting good heart health as well as weight loss. Cardio includes anything that gets your heart rate up and pumping above your normal resting rate. To find out what your working heart rate is you must first know your resting heart rate. The best time to take your resting heart rate is first thing in the morning. It should be in the range of 60-80 beats per minute. To take your working heart rate, take your pulse on the inside of your wrist, on the thumb side. Use the tips of your first two fingers (not your other thumb) to press lightly over the blood vessels on your wrist leading to your thumb. Count your pulse for ten seconds and multiply by six to find your beats per minute. Your target heart rate during exercise should stay between 50 to 85 percent of your maximum heart rate. (Your maximum heart rate is about 220 minus your age.)[4]

Many people associate cardio with a treadmill or elliptical machine, but you can actually get a good cardio workout by playing your favorite sport, dancing, or even lifting weights.

Interval Training

When people will ask me what type of cardio workouts I like, I always respond with "lifting weights." You see, what I like to do is called interval weight training. This is a high intensity workout that includes focused and intense lifting that keeps your heart rate pumping. It is then followed by a short break to slow your heart down. Doing this over the course of 50 minutes is a great way to work both your muscles and your heart. The reason I prefer this method is because when you do some other forms of cardio exercise, though it will be good for your heart, your body will stop burning calories as soon as you are done exercising. When you add weights to your cardio exercise in the form of interval training, you help your body build your muscles, and those muscles will help burn calories and fat for the rest of your day. To be honest, I also have a tendency to get bored quickly if I am on a treadmill or an elliptical, but interval training keeps my mind and body engaged at the same time.

I generally split up my workouts so that I am focusing on certain parts of my body each day, and I spread these workouts throughout the week. For example, one day I will lift weights that focus on my chest and biceps. The next time I will work on my back and legs, and a few days later I will work my shoulders and triceps. I also like to incorporate some abdominal workouts twice a week to make sure my core is staying firm. You can find more information online regarding which workouts will help you to work certain areas of your body. If you are like me, I encourage you to give interval training a try. While there will always be times when you have to mentally push through a workout, I think exercise should be enjoyable and exciting overall.

Crossfit

Crossfit has really taken off over the past few years. It was developed to give you a full body workout that combines elements of cardio, weightlifting, gymnastics, and core training.[5] It's important to note that one should be careful when beginning crossfit. Don't be afraid to ask the coach to walk you through how to do each workout properly. Most coaches will be more than happy to help you and answer any questions that you may have, which can help to protect you from injury.

Swimming

As children, many of us looked forward to the summer days when we could splash around in a pool for hours! At the time we didn't realize that it was giving us a good workout. As adults, many of us don't actually swim in the pool anymore but just lounge next to it with a book or iced tea. Let us take a lesson from the kids! Swimming is a wonderful way to add cardio—even muscle tone—to your body. I know a lady who weighed 480 pounds; she was desperate to lose weight. She knew that any physical activity was going to be hard on her body, especially her joints, but instead of feeling defeated, she decided to begin swimming because it would give her a good workout while alleviating joint pressure. I was so impressed by her determination. When you submerge your body in water up to your neck, you only have to bear 10 percent of your body weight because the water carries the other 90 percent. If you have arthritis, this could be a great exercise option for you as well.[6]

Stretching

One thing that I am intentional about doing before my workout is stretching. I know that there are differing opinions about whether you should stretch before or after you work out, but I personally find that I do better if I stretch beforehand. Whether before or after—just stretch! It is crucial for your body because it starts the flow of blood to your muscles, which in turn will help you move better. I personally seem to carry a lot of tension in my hips, so making sure I stretch that area regularly helps relieve pain and prevent injury. Many people don't like stretching because they are frustrated by how inflexible they feel. I think the key is to start off slow. Flexibility comes with time, and don't stretch your muscles too hard because that can lead to injury.

Pilates

Pilates is a great form of exercise because it focuses and challenges your core while also working other parts of your body as well. Many gyms offer Pilates classes, and you can find some great ones on YouTube as well.

These are just a few ideas to help you in your fitness journey. The goal is to find something that you enjoy so that exercise doesn't become a chore. Whether it's lifting weights for an hour at the gym, going for a bike ride, or pressing "play" to work out with a YouTube Pilates video, just do it!

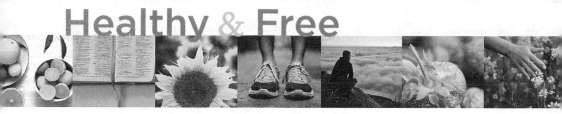
4.4

Eating Clean

Ahh, food. I love good food, and I love to eat. I am a self-proclaimed foodie! Thankfully, my husband is a food lover too, and we often find ourselves searching for new restaurants where the food on the menu not only appeals to our taste buds but is also good for our bodies.

People are often surprised when they hear how passionate I am about food and especially when I tell them that I eat a lot. In fact, over the years, one of the secrets I have learned to help maintain a healthy weight for my size and my age is to eat plenty of fresh foods. Through my own experience, and watching countless friends struggle, I have come to believe that one of the systemic problems in the diet industry is the persistent overemphasis on low-calorie eating or what I call "glorified starvation diets." As many can attest, the sad reality is that most diets just do not work! In addition to the emphasis on low calories, which I will elaborate on later, I believe one of the main reasons for this is found in our thinking. The prevailing mindset of a person who goes on a diet is thinking that once they reach their goal weight they will be free to go back to eating the way that they used to before they started the diet. Usually, they then begin to

73

obsess about all the food that is "not allowed" on their diet until they finally crack from the pressure and eat the forbidden items. For some, this can take the form of binge eating that can last for days, weeks, and even months. Before they know it, all the weight that they lost through dieting has been regained, and sadly, sometimes they will end up with more unwanted pounds than before they started. This can lead to dark feelings of depression and defeat—even shame that once again they have failed. This is not God's heart for us.

A further drawback to fad dieting is that it can indirectly exacerbate a weight problem. While the promises of quick weight loss are appealing, in reality it can often lead to muscle loss. This is a serious setback for one's health because, as we discussed in the chapter on exercise, muscle burns fat. Losing it not only causes other physical problems, but it makes a weight-loss journey much more difficult.

Another reason why dieting is ineffective is because it often leads to a chronic, yo-yo cycle of gaining and losing weight, and our bodies don't respond well to periods of chronic hunger followed by feasting. If you are constantly forcing yourself to eat less or denying yourself the foods that you're craving, then you can cause your body to think that food is limited and literally "trick" your body into believing that it needs to switch into calorie-storing mode, as if you were living in a famine when food is scarce.

When I say "dieting," I mean the act of forcibly trying to control either the quantity or quality of what you are eating, which is a form of starvation. Jon Gabriel, author of the *The Gabriel Method,* argues that this practice can make your body think that it needs to carry around extra fat so that it activates what he calls the FAT programs. He writes,

> FAT programs operate as signals to the body to retain fat. Food additives, mental and emotional threats, medications, radiation, nutritional starvation, emotional obesity (as in the case of abuse), fear of scarcity, mental starvation, dysfunctional beliefs, and chronic yo-yo dieting are all FAT programs.[1]

I want to encourage people to recognize these triggers, stop dieting, and start nourishing their bodies with healthy, organic, living foods.

I once had two women come to me seeking advice on how to lose weight. My first question to them was, "How much do you eat?" They both told me that they hardly ate anything at all, so they were puzzled as to why they weren't losing weight. I knew right away that this was their problem. Our bodies need food to burn fat. I gave them an assignment to eat 200–250 calorie meals every two hours, and to make sure they were made up of healthy, clean proteins, fat, and carbs. Within two weeks, both ladies came back to me in shock over how much weight they had begun to lose. Isn't it interesting how they seemed to gain weight when they starved themselves, but lost weight when they ate every two hours! You see, when you starve your body, your brain tells it to store all your fat because it knows that it's not getting enough in your diet. Once you begin to eat good, healthy, clean foods, your body will respond and will work for you.

What to Eat?

Let's first define the term "clean eating." Clean eating means that you consume foods that are pure and true to their natural form. This includes an abundance of foods like fruit, vegetables, healthy proteins, and good fats. Clean eating helps you eliminate processed foods like refined sugar, salt, and flour from your diet. In addition, a lot of the foods that Americans consume contains Genetically Modified Organisms, or GMOs. I don't know about you, but just the sound of that makes me want to avoid putting them into my body! Whenever something is classified as a GMO, it means that it has been altered at the genetic level. It may also have been pumped full of hormones, pesticides, antibiotics, and chemicals. I will get into this topic later in this chapter, but as the old saying goes, "If you can't read or pronounce the ingredients, don't eat it!" These certainly don't qualify as clean eating.

We've covered the basics regarding how to eat clean by avoiding unhealthy ingredients and processed foods as much as possible. Now I want to tell you about some of the science behind these choices, starting with macronutrients. Macronutrients provide calories or energy for our bodies.[2] They can be broken down into three categories: fats, proteins, and carbs. It's important to have all of these because each plays an important role in keeping your body healthy.

How much of each category does a person need? I can tell you right off the bat that everybody is different. First, you need to figure out what your ideal caloric intake should be. To start, take your body weight. Next, you will want to look over the following list and select the number that best reflects your lifestyle. For example, if you weigh 130 pounds and you work in a sedentary office job and you do not exercise, your lifestyle would fall under number 11. Multiply 130 by 11 and you will get 1,430. This number should be your daily caloric intake.

These descriptions will help you find the right multiplier:

- Multiply by 11 if you have a sedentary job in which you get little physical activity.

- Multiply by 12 if you have a relatively active job (postman, standing receptionist at a front desk, cleaner, etc.), or if you have a sedentary job but you work out two or three days a week.

- Multiply by 13 if you have an active job and you train two or three times a week, or a sedentary job and you train at an intense level four to six times a week.

- Multiply by 14 if you have an active job and you train at an intense level four to six times a week, or if you are an athlete and you train every day or multiple times a day.

Once you have figured out your ideal caloric intake, you can then begin to figure out how many of those calories should consist of each of the macronutrients: proteins, fats, and carbs.

Protein

Protein should be a fundamental part of your diet and figuring out how much you need is pretty simple. It's recommended that you eat one gram of protein for every pound that you weigh. So if you weigh 130 pounds, you will want to eat 130 grams of protein per day. I know that for those who are athletic, extremely muscular, or overweight this may seem like a great deal, and eating that much each day might be a challenge. If that is you, I recommend that you take a look at your protein intake and just try to increase it. Protein is one of our main body builders. Everything from muscles to hormones, enzymes, and antibodies is made up of protein. Protein can also help prevent blood clots, create fluid balance, and promote transportation of vital substances throughout the body. It can also be used for energy when our intake of carbohydrates and fat is low.[3]

When you choose proteins for your diet, try to stick to high-quality, organic sources such as lean red meats, poultry, fish, cottage cheese, milk, natural nut butters, peas, broccoli, organic corn, chickpeas, spinach, and kale. There are also many good protein powders that can help supplement your protein intake. I use a vegan protein powder made of peas, hemp, and cranberry.

Fats

Despite what you may have heard or read about fats, they are not all the same. What many people refer to as "good fats" happen to be great for your health. In the 90s, low-fat diets became all the rage and people began looking for products that contained little or no fat. Unfortunately, when food manufacturers reduce fat, they tend to replace it with sugar, which, as we all know, can lead to health problems. In fact, eating good and healthy fats in the right amounts can actually aid weight loss as well as improve metabolism. Good fats are vital to your brain. Here's why:

Approximately 60 percent of your brain matter consists of fats that create all the cell membranes in your body.…. The good fat in your brain matter creates all the cell membranes in your body! If your diet is loaded with bad fats, your brain can only make low-quality nerve cell membranes that don't function well; if your diet provides the essential, good fats, your brain cells can manufacture higher-quality nerve cell membranes and influence positively your nerve cells' ability to function at their peak capacity.…

Thus, it's important to choose foods that offer the essential fatty acids your body and brain need. Unfortunately, even good fats are a very concentrated source of energy, providing more than double the amount of calories in one gram of carbohydrate or protein, which is why it's important to choose the healthy fats and to eat them in moderation.[4]

You need between .3 and .6 grams of fat per pound of body weight. This should largely be based on personal preference. As long as you are eating a minimum of .3 and not exceeding .6, you are doing well. To determine what your ideal intake should be, think of your favorite types of foods. If you tend to enjoy fattier foods such as cheese, bacon, nuts, and rich desserts, then I'd suggest you aim for .5 to .6 grams per pound of body weight. If, on the other hand you are more of a "carbo-holic" who craves breads, pasta, chips, and pretzels, then aim for .3 to .4 grams of fat per pound. Doing it this way will allow you to indulge as well as enjoy your favorite foods more often, and will help you stick to your eating plan. Your carb and fat intake will be inversely proportional, meaning the higher one is, the lower the other will be. Therefore, you can reduce your fat in order to consume more carbs and vice versa. The only exception to this is if you are an athlete who is focused on performance and need to recover quickly after a workout—then you should keep your carb intake moderate to high regardless of fat intake. If you rarely train or only engage in light exercise, then your carb tolerance is likely to be lower so you should set your fat intake toward the higher end of the scale.

As with any other food group, you want to make sure that you are eating good, clean fats, which your body can easily utilize. There are many good fats which will help your body as you develop a healthy lifestyle. Foods such as wild salmon, cod, nuts, seeds, avocados (which are a "complete" food meaning they contain fat, carbs, and protein), and oils such as flaxseed oil, olive oil, fish oils, and coconut oil are good fats. Years ago, we were told to stay away from coconut oil, but now there is new research, which demonstrates that it is actually good for you and that using small amounts of coconut oil can actually help you lose weight.[5]

Carbohydrates

Carbs have been given a bad rap in today's diet industry, which has resulted in many crash diets where carbs are eliminated altogether in the hopes of losing weight quickly. Often people will go as long as they can without carbs only to crash and begin bingeing. This is because carbs provide our bodies with energy and the lack of them will actually increase cravings for sugar and other junk foods because your body wants to satisfy its need for fuel. A great tool to find what your daily macronutrient goals should be, go to www.iifym.com and use their macro calculator.

You will want to stick with complex carbohydrates that are commonly found in vegetables, wholemeal breads, and cereals. Foods such as spinach, yams, broccoli, beans, brown rice, quinoa, zucchini, lentils, skim milk, whole grains, and many other leguminous plants and vegetables are good sources of healthy carbs. For breads, I'd recommend brands such as Ezekiel bread or Manna bread, or any good company that also uses sprouted grains. There are also many great Paleo breads that you can find on the market or better yet—make some at home for yourself and your family.

Organic vs. Conventional Foods

By now, many of us know that it is always better to eat organic. The reason for this is that conventional fruit or vegetables (otherwise known as the unlabeled, standard produce found in your average supermarket) are loaded with harmful chemicals and additives to help preserve them. Our food today is filled with these artificial additions as well as growth hormones and antibiotics. Sadly, the list goes on. I don't know about you, but when I think about what is actually in our food (not to mention what it has been sprayed with) I feel very motivated to buy organic food whenever I can. Conventional fruit and vegetables have been grown in soil that has been depleted of the minerals that our bodies need. I recommend that everyone watch the documentary *Food Inc.* because it gives you an inside look into what the big food industries are doing to our food.[6] It is a good but sobering film because it reveals how unhealthy our basic foods have become.

I was once in one of our local grocery stores looking for organic apples only to discover that they were sold out. I approached the produce manager to inquire when they would be restocked, and he responded by trying to convince me to purchase conventional apples, claiming that they were just as good as the organic ones. I politely smiled and walked away. I know too much about the difference between organic and conventional farming—not to mention the difference in taste!—to have followed his advice. If you have ever compared a conventional apple to an organic apple, you will notice that the conventional apple is bland. This is because the soil where it was grown has been depleted from minerals and nutrients over time, causing the food to lose flavor. When you grow food in rich, organic soil, you will get a much finer product that will taste good as well as contain the nutrients that your body needs for good health.

People often ask me, "How can I afford to eat organic?" The way I see it is that you can pay for your food now or you can pay the doctor, and the price for poor health, later. We now have more organic options available to us. Farmer's markets have become more popular, and a "go-to" option for many families who want to buy locally grown food that is full of life instead of chemicals. I know many people who have begun to grow their own fruit and vegetables or who have joined a community garden, which saves money in the long run. In our community, several families split the cost of buying a side of beef together (100 percent grass finished), which lowers the price per pound. The Internet is also a great tool for economizing because you can order from excellent organic companies at a discount or in bulk, all without having to leave the comfort of your home.

If you are on a really tight budget and can only afford a few organic items, I always recommend starting with milk and eggs. Cows and chickens who are raised conventionally are pumped full of chemicals and hormones throughout their lives. Sadly, their milk and eggs are going to be filled with the same additives. Just making the simple change to organic milk and eggs can provide a huge benefit to your health, especially for your growing children (who will benefit the most from hormone-free dairy products).

As far as produce is concerned, here is a list of foods that contain above average amounts of pesticides. When deciding whether to buy organic or conventional, the following should be on your list of organic foods to choose first: apples, cherries, bell peppers, peaches, nectarines, potatoes, raspberries, strawberries, spinach, celery, grapes, and pears. Foods that are usually lower in pesticides are bananas, onions, eggplant, broccoli, watermelon, cabbage, avocado, tomatoes, mangoes, papaya, peas, pineapple, corn, kiwi, and asparagus.[7] Do remember, these foods still contain some pesticides so if you can, buy organic and make sure the label says "USDA Certified Organic." There are many ways to find organic foods that you can afford. Sure, it might take a bit of effort on your part, but the benefits far outweigh the sacrifice.

GMO Foods

As if the previous section didn't give us enough reason to want to buy organic, I am going to give you yet another reason. GMO's. Three small letters that come with one big problem. What does GMO mean? As I mentioned earlier it stands for "Genetically Modified Organism." They are plants or animals created through the gene-splicing techniques of biotechnology (also called genetic engineering or GE). This experimental technology merges DNA from different species, creating unstable combinations of plant, animal, bacterial, and viral genes that do not occur in nature or in traditional crossbreeding.[8] In the United States, more than 80 percent of many major crops are grown from genetically engineered seed and about 70 percent of processed foods contain GMOs.[9]

There is currently a big fight in the US regarding the labeling of GMOs in our food. The polls tell us that people want to know what is in their food, but big industries have the resources to stop the labeling of GMOs through supporting the powerful biotech lobby. So far they have succeeded in keeping mandatory labeling of this information from the public.[10]

By purchasing organic food labeled "GMO free," you are protecting yourself from possible harm that GMO products may cause. There is so much research yet to be done in this area. By buying organic, non-GMO food you not only reduce potential risk to your health, but you also you receive the benefits of nutrient-dense food.

Sugar

As I mentioned earlier in this book, I used to be a hard-core sugar addict. I know that many struggle when they are trying to "come off" sugar, and I am not surprised. Did you know that sugar has actually been proven to be more addictive than hard drugs such as cocaine?[11] When I was breaking free from my sugar addiction, I had to find alternatives. I loved the taste of sugary treats, but I knew that eating refined, white sugar and high fructose corn syrup (which, by the way, is in many processed foods) would make me sick; they were actually like poison to my body. So, I started on a search to find healthy alternatives so that I could keep my body and my sweet tooth both happy and healthy. What I learned is that you need to find a low-glycemic sugar that will not spike or disrupt your blood sugar level. In order for it not to affect your blood sugar level, the sweetening agent that you use needs to be 55 or below on the glycemic scale. Here is a list of low-glycemic sugars and where they fall:[12]

- Natural Maple Syrup: 54

- Natural Honey: 50

- Natural Yacon Syrup: 1

- Coconut Palm Sugar: 35

- Stevia: 0

If you use Stevia, remember that in its original form it comes from a plant, so when it is turned into a powder or liquid consistency it must be processed. Therefore, always read the labels to make sure it is pure Stevia, that it hasn't had corn syrup added to it, and find a good, organic brand. I have done some research on Stevia and I have to admit, it gets mixed reviews. Some say that it causes infertility while others say that it helps promote fertility.[13] My suggestion is that if you prefer to use Stevia, consider incorporating other sweeteners into your diet as well. Anything that has zero calories can be questionable, so I make sure to alternate between Stevia and honey.[14]

One last tip on the subject of sugar—avoid artificial sweeteners. Aspartame and Splenda have been linked to numerous diseases and conditions such as migraines, depression, memory loss, and even brain cancer.[15] Once, when I went to see my massage therapist I mentioned to her that I was feeling extremely achy in my body. Her first question was if I used Splenda. A little confused, I told her yes. (This was during the time when I was trying to overcome my sugar addiction and I used Splenda as a substitute.) She suggested that I stop using it, explaining that when Splenda is ingested our bodies don't know what to do with it, since it is a foreign substance, so it gets stored in our joints. I took her advice, and within a very short amount of time I noticed that my aches were completely gone. Similarly, I have a friend who had gone to see a colonics doctor after struggling for years with digestive issues. As the doctor massaged and examined her stomach she asked if my friend used a lot of Splenda. (She was like me and thought that Splenda was healthy, so she was ingesting quite a bit.) Her doctor advised her to stop, because in her experience, it could turn into a stone-like substance in the digestive tract, potentially leading to different types of digestion problems. There have also been reports that Splenda can destroy up to 50 percent of the good bacteria in your gut.[16] After looking into it, I decided to stop using it altogether. I encourage you to do your own research, looking at both sides of the controversy, and then you can decide what you think will be best for your health.

The Power of Superfoods

"Superfoods" are powerful additions to nutrition that provide high doses of antioxidants, polyphenols, vitamins, and minerals.[17] I love adding superfoods to my meals because they are healthy and taste great at the same time. Here are some superfoods that you can consider trying:

- Chia Seeds: Chia seeds have been used for hundreds of years for their ability to provide stamina and strength. It has been said that the Aztec warriors ate them before going into battle to help give them endurance.[18] They are a great source of antioxidants, fiber, magnesium, fat, and protein.[19]

- Gogi berries: Gogi berries pack quite the nutritional punch when it comes to health benefits. The Gogi berry has been used in Chinese medicine for hundreds of years. It has a high dose of vitamin C, contains more carotenoids than any other food, has 21 trace minerals, and is high in fiber.[20] It has also been said to help promote mental wellness by alleviating depression and promoting healthy sleep.[21] If you are taking blood-thinning medication, consult with your doctor before adding Gogi berries to your diet.

- Hemp Seeds: These have been said to be the most nutritious seeds in the world. Not only are hemp seeds a complete protein (5 grams of protein per two tablespoon serving), but they also help promote weight loss, increased energy, lowered cholesterol and blood pressure, reduced inflammation, improvement in circulation and immune system as well as being a type of natural blood sugar control.[22]

- Flax Seeds: These small but mighty seeds are a great source of omega-3 fatty acids, which help reduce and prevent inflammation in our bodies. They are also high in fiber, magnesium and manganese, which promotes healthy digestion. Flax seed is a great source of lignans, which convert in our intestines to substances that help balance female hormones.[23] If you are like me, and you don't care for the texture of flaxseeds, you can purchase them ground. Then you can add them into smoothies, baking, and cooking,

- Kale: Kale seems to be the most popular superfood right now, which makes sense considering all the health benefits it provides. It is high in fiber (2.5 grams in one cup), vitamins A, C, K, and folate, which is a form of a vitamin B that supports brain development.[24]

This is just a short list of superfoods. I love researching these treasures and finding all the benefits that God has placed into each one. Don't be afraid to go online, do some research yourself, and try new and exciting foods in the process.

Gluten

I am sure that most of us by now have heard about gluten. The questions that everyone is asking are, "Why are so many people choosing food that is gluten-free? Is this just a fad or is there a real reason for concern?"

First of all, let's talk about what gluten is. It is a binding protein that is typically found in wheat, barley, and rye products. Gluten can also be found in many whole-grain foods related to wheat, including bulgur, farro, kamut, spelt, and triticale. It is used to give bread texture, help it to rise, and is used as a thickening agent in many sauces and soups.[25] Gluten has been around for centuries so my question is, "Why is it that so many more people are gluten sensitive now than a few years ago?"

Here are two thoughts on this subject. Scientists suggest that there may be more problems with gluten today because people eat greater amounts of processed wheat products like pastas and baked goods than in decades past. Not only are people consuming more gluten-saturated products today, but those items that use gluten have a much higher content than they used to.

Another theory regarding the rise in gluten allergies suggests that it is a result of the way it is made today. In the 1950s, scientists began crossbreeding wheat to make it heartier, shorter, and easier to grow. This was the basis of the Green Revolution that boosted wheat harvests worldwide. Yet the new crossbred gluten in our wheat may now have become the very thing that is troublesome for many people. This also may have been a contributing factor in the rise of the newly labeled condition called "gluten sensitivity."

Early in my journey, I made the decision to go on a 60-day fast from all gluten. I found that I did much better without it. My digestive processes were more consistent and I felt that I had more energy as well. Signs for me of being gluten sensitive were bloating, gas, upset stomach, and brain fog. Because I now know what it feels like to be off of gluten, I can immediately tell when I have accidentally eaten something that contains it. For me, the benefits of being off gluten far outweigh the loss of a piece of bread. There are some great gluten-free bread options available too for those who just cannot bear the thought of sacrificing bread. Personally, I try to keep my diet grain-free so I don't eat gluten-free bread. The fact that gluten-free bread tends to have little to no nutrients in it makes it an easy decision for me. From time to time, I will try sprouted organic bread, which doesn't tend to upset my stomach as much.

Some people have what is called celiac disease, which is an auto-immune disorder that causes their bodies to be intolerant to gluten in any form. When people with celiac disease eat gluten their body mounts an immune response that attacks the small intestine. These attacks damage the villi, the small, fingerlike projections lining the small intestine that promote nutrient absorption. When the villi become damaged, nutrients cannot be absorbed properly into the body.[26] While not a high percentage of people suffer from celiac disease, there are many who have gluten sensitivity, which can have some similar symptoms.

Interestingly, I have seen many people who are obese go off gluten, and immediately start losing weight. One of our pastors was praying for a woman who had fibromyalgia. While praying, he felt he needed to tell her to go off gluten. This is *not* something that he would normally tell a person to do, but she felt it was right and agreed. Since she did it, she has been fine.

If, after reading this, you are wondering whether some of your health problems might be a result of gluten, I would suggest that you go on a gluten-free fast for 60 days and see how you feel. Remember to always read the labels of the foods you choose, and be careful not to eat sauces and dressings if they are not labeled because they contain gluten. Many restaurants have become aware of the issues surrounding gluten, and now offer menus with gluten-free options.

Healthy Lifestyle Options

While I don't agree with diets and dieting, I do believe that there are lifestyles and patterns of healthy eating which work for some people. The following are several which have benefitted me or other people that I know and trust. They may not be right for you, but they may spark new, creative ideas, and operate as a type of general guide to new approaches. Your healthcare professional is also an ally, and should be consulted in any major dietary change. At the same time, as I have maintained since the beginning of this book, God is your guide, your partner, and your friend. He knows every detail of your body and He will work with you more effectively than any book or person. As Scripture says: "Whether you turn to the right or to the left, your ears will hear a voice behind you saying, 'This is the way, walk in it'" (Isa. 30:21, NIV).

Paleo diet (as in paleolithic or caveman)

This style of eating omits legumes, grains, and most dairy (although some people choose to eat organic butter and ghee from grass-fed cows). Many find success with this lifestyle primarily because it eradicates processed foods from one's diet, which in turn eliminates many added chemicals and preservatives. The goal is to eat all food in its raw, natural state. Organic, cooked poultry, red meat, and pork are all permissible. Organic fruits and vegetables can be eaten in limitless amounts (but remember that fruit contains sugar so if you are trying to lose weight perhaps eat less of it). In regard to potatoes, most "paleos" only eat sweet potatoes and yams. They are higher in calories and carbs, so they are good to eat right after a workout to replenish your glycogen levels.[27] People who are following a paleo approach to healthy eating enjoy nuts and seeds (excluding peanuts, which are considered a legume and not a nut) because they are a great source of healthy fats and proteins. Also, good quality, organic, cold-pressed oils like olive, avocado, and coconut oil are encouraged as additional forms of healthy fats. Wild fish is a good source of protein that is usually safer to consume than farm-raised fish, which often contains mercury and other toxins. Organic omega-3 eggs can be another great option for someone pursuing this style of eating. The paleo diet has been a really successful approach to eating for people who have gluten and grain intolerance, celiac disease, or autoimmune disorders.

Vegetarian diet

A vegetarian diet is rich in fruits, vegetables, nuts, seeds, and legumes. Vegetarians refrain from eating animal meat, but some will allow dairy and eggs. (Vegans are vegetarians who eliminate all animal products from their diets, including dairy products and eggs.) Important considerations for vegetarians and vegans is first to be careful not to overload their diets with too many grains, and to make sure that they eat plenty of protein from the sources available to them.

GAPS (Gut and Psychology Syndrome) diet

This nutritional approach was created by Dr. Natasha Campbell-McBride after raising a child with learning disabilities. Recommended foods are organic eggs, fresh meats, fish, shellfish, fresh fruits, vegetables, nuts and seeds, garlic and olive oil. This diet encourages eating as many raw vegetables as you can on the theory that the enzymes in uncooked vegetables can help digest food while healing the digestive tract. The GAPS diet encourages people to eat fruit on its own because the digestive tract handles it differently than other foods; the theory is that fruit can cause pain and discomfort when eaten with other foods, so it is recommended as an in-between-meals snack. Natural fats are recommended also, such as olive and coconut oil, ghee, and nuts. This diet also includes a high amount of fermented foods such as sauerkraut, yogurt, and kefir since they are believed to play a vital role in keeping the digestive tract healthy. For more information, you can purchase Dr. Campbell-McBride's book, *Gut and Psychology Syndrome*.[28] This approach to eating is frequently recommended for people who have stomach and digestive problems such as IBS and "leaky gut" syndrome, and has been used as a supportive diet for people dealing with autism, mood and mental disorders.

Mediterranean diet

Dr. Ancel Keys, an American scientist, created this approach after living abroad in Italy in the 1950s. He noticed that the people in Southern Europe seemed to have less disease and lived more vibrant, healthy lives than people in other parts of the world.[29] He advocated a very simple diet consisting of vegetables, fruits, nuts, seeds, legumes, potatoes, whole grain breads, herbs, spices, fish, seafood, and extra virgin olive oil, with poultry, eggs, cheese, and yogurt eaten in moderation. His goal was to simplify food choices without sacrificing flavor. Dr. Keys discouraged the use of sweetened beverages, added sugars, processed meat, refined grains, refined oils, and other highly processed foods. Because of its heart-healthy options, this diet is recommended particularly for people with heart conditions or heart disease, but anyone can follow this methodology.

Eat Right for Your [Blood] Type

Peter D'Adamo is the best-known proponent of this approach to healthy living. He believes that your ideal diet is determined by your blood type, which could explain why certain foods are good for some while intolerable for others. I used the blood type regimen for a while, and I felt better than I ever have before. However, I found that I was not able to commit to it as a lifestyle because there were certain foods that I loved too much to give up.[30]

Here is a very basic breakdown: (1) **Type O blood:** People with type O blood are thought to do best on high-protein diets (featuring lean meats such as chicken, fish, and turkey) that go light on grains, beans, and dairy. (2) **Type A blood:** People with type A blood seem to do well on more plant-based diets (fresh, organic fruits and vegetables with legumes, and whole grains). (3) **Type B blood:** Those with type B blood are encouraged to avoid corn, wheat, buckwheat, lentils, tomatoes, peanuts, and sesame seeds. D'Adamo believes that even chicken can be problematic for this blood type. He encourages eating green vegetables, eggs, certain meats, and low-fat dairy. (4) **Type AB blood:** According to D'Adamo, type ABs need a diet that is more focused on organic seafood, dairy, and green vegetables as they tend to have lower levels of stomach acids than the other blood types. He also recommends staying away from meats as they can require more "digestive strength."

Make Your Own Choices

These healthy lifestyle choices are only a few of the options available to you out of many. There are many fad diets that, in my opinion, cause more harm than good. In contrast, the ones listed above may help with giving you some ideas to get started on your journey to wellness. In my own life, I try to follow the 80/20 rule which means that 80 percent of what I eat consists of raw foods (fruits and vegetables), while 20 percent is so-called "dead food," which means foods that have been cooked. Whatever path you decide to take, remember that grace is the key when changing your eating habits.

I am aware that I just gave you a lot of information in this chapter, but I don't want you to feel overwhelmed. Rather, my heart is for you to feel empowered. As with anything, start small and simple. Some may need to just start by adding more fruits and vegetables to their diets, while others may feel more inclined to do an entire lifestyle change at once. However you do it, always allow yourself grace to try things out, ease into changes slowly, take time, and change your mind. Remember, this is journey and not a race.

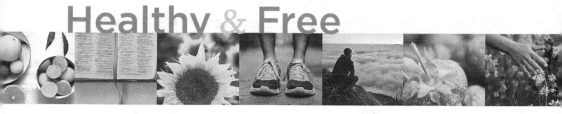

4.5

Detoxing for a Better Life

Recently, as I was studying this subject again, I began to marvel over the way that God created our bodies in such intricate detail. He made every tissue, every organ, all our nerves and blood to work together in perfect harmony. Since He specifically designed the body to self-clean and detox itself, you might ask the question, "If our bodies are supposed to detox naturally, why then do we have to do anything extra to help them in the process?" The sad reality is that the environments we live in are often full of toxins. There are pesticides in our foods, chemicals in our cleaning products, and even the air we breathe has 187 known toxins in it.[1] We can go about our day-to-day lives choosing a healthy lifestyle, yet still come into contact with toxins in the air we breathe, the foods we eat, the water we drink, our cleaning supplies, makeup products, lotions and facial cleansers, the mattresses we sleep on, the clothes we wear, the carpets in our homes, and even in some of the supplements we take.

These toxins can be very harmful if they continue to build up in your system. An overload of toxins in your body has been linked to weight gain, cancer, Alzheimer's, autism, diabetes, fatigue, heart disease, allergies, candida, and infertility.[2] Dr. Mark Hyman says, "If you are struggling to lose weight despite eating well and exercising…toxins may be interfering with your body's metabolism."[3] So it seems that detoxing your body could play a very important role in keeping your body healthy.

God designed your body to detox naturally by neutralizing, transforming, and processing unwanted materials and toxins. Therefore, when we talk about detoxification we are talking about improving and optimizing the existing functions of our body's own detoxification system. We can do this by decreasing the amount of toxins that we put into our bodies while at the same time supporting their detoxification and elimination systems with the nutrients that they need in order to function properly. In doing this, I believe that we can optimize our health.[4]

Having said that, I must add that there are diverse opinions among healthcare providers regarding this subject. Some believe that we should not do anything to assist our bodies in detoxing because, as I said above, our bodies detox themselves. Some say you only need to detox for a few days while others suggest detoxing for a week. Others feel that because there is an overload of toxins in our world, it is impossible for our bodies to fully detox on their own. The question follows, "If I do detox, what should I do, and how long should I do it?"

The vast array of information can all become very confusing and overwhelming, so my advice is this: Listen to your body. You know your body better than anybody else and only you can really sense when it feels "off." As always, talk these decisions over with your healthcare provider and remember to rely on the Holy Spirit as your Guide. I am very sensitive to what is going on in my body because I've taught myself to listen to it, and I can tell almost immediately when it needs some assistance through detoxing. I will usually begin to feel sluggish and heavy, like something just isn't right.

The Signs of Toxicity

As I said, your body will probably tell you when something is off balance. A lot of times, people are so used to feeling sick that they don't realize their symptoms are actually a cry for help. Here are some signs that your body may need a detox:

- **Fatigue**: In general, feeling tired isn't necessarily abnormal especially with busy schedules and lack of sleep. However, if you struggle with extreme fatigue and feel that it takes every ounce of energy to just get out of bed, you may be due for a detox. This is normally not because your body is worn out from having to keep you awake and alive, but rather because it may be overworking from trying to eliminate toxins that are overloading your system. When they reach this point of exhaustion, many people reach for more coffee or energy drinks, which only add to the problem. Toxins can cause your immune system to get worn down which may lead to repetitive illness, which can then lead to more fatigue—an unfortunate cycle.

- **Weight fluctuation**: If you are eating a clean, healthy diet as well as exercising, but you still can't seem to lose weight, then an overload of toxins could be the culprit. The main focus of a body saturated with toxins becomes the need to eliminate them, which means that weight loss will be last on its list of priorities.

- **Halitosis**: Bad breath is often not a symptom of poor oral hygiene but rather of an imbalance in the digestive system. Some link halitosis to the liver which is the main organ that eliminates toxins. Sometimes people will use gum to try to mask their bad breath, but most brands of chewing gum on the market are

95

loaded with more toxins like artificial sweeteners, which means that the attempt to mask the problem may make it worse.

- **Constipation**: This is a condition that we all want to avoid. Not only does it make us uncomfortable and irritable, but it can also cause upset stomachs, headaches, muscle pains, and fatigue. When an excess of toxins gets caught in the intestines, it then can cause your digestive track to get clogged up. My advice is to eliminate all processed foods and to make sure you eat plenty of living foods. Drink good, clean water to help keep your digestive system regular.

- **Smell sensitivity**: Being sensitive to smell isn't just for pregnant women! Many people actually experience a smell sensitivity when their bodies become overloaded with toxins. Our bodies communicate with us and one of the ways they do is by making us sensitive to chemical smells when they have had enough. If you have frequent headaches or nausea due to scents, then your body may be trying to tell you something.

- **Muscle pain**: Have you ever woken up sore but couldn't figure out why because you couldn't recall doing any strenuous activity? This could be because your body is beginning to store extra toxins in your muscles because it can't expel them.

- **Skin reactions:** Acne, rashes, puffy eyes, eczema, and psoriasis are all signs that you may have an excess of toxins in your body. Make sure that you take an inventory of your skincare and makeup products, many of which have chemicals and parabens that can get absorbed into your system through your skin.

What's Next?

If some of these symptoms relate to you, you may wonder what to do next. We all have major organs in our bodies that are designed to work together and help keep our body clean. These major organs include the stomach, small intestine, pancreas, lungs, large intestine (colon), liver, kidneys, heart, brain, and skin. As we discussed, when these organs are overloaded with toxins we can feel fatigued, sluggish, and even ill.

First step, we will go over the roles that these organs play and see how we can assist them in the detox process.

The Colon

Let me start off by saying that talking about the colon is awkward and humorous at the same time; I admit I laughed a lot while researching this topic. Let's be real—everybody poops. So for the moment, let's set aside the awkwardness of this subject so that we can pay attention to our health. Naturopathic doctors will tell you to begin with the colon (or "gut") when you consider detoxing. Health care professionals call the gut "the second brain," since it plays such an important role in the overall health of the body.[5] It has also been said that 90 percent of disease starts in the colon. I have known people who had severe allergies, but once they began colon-cleansing, their allergies completely disappeared! Such information has convinced me to make it a point to keep my colon cleansed at all times.

A sign of a healthy colon is having two or three bowel movements a day. That can be a shocking number considering a lot of Americans only have two or three bowel movements a week! A baby's digestion gives us a good example of gut health. Any parent can attest to just how much a tiny baby can poop. In fact, our bodies were designed to poop after every time we eat, and that keeps a person's gut healthy.

Not only should you pay attention to the number of times you poop, but also to the way it looks. Your bowel movement should look like a snake. It should be smooth and soft. There is debate about whether your stool should sink or float, but I believe that either is fine as long as you are defecating regularly.[6]

A few ways to make sure that you are moving your bowels regularly include drinking plenty of water, consuming healthy oils, and eating lots of fiber. It is recommended that women consume between 21 and 25 grams of fiber per day and men between 30 and 38 grams.[7] There are plenty of fiber supplements on the market that can help you to make sure that you get enough fiber. However, I believe that it's always best to get your fiber from healthy, fiber-containing foods such as fruits and vegetables as well as chia and flax seeds. You can also get your daily dose of oils from foods like avocados, olive oil, fish oil, coconut oil, flaxseed oil, and hemp seed oil. They will lubricate your intestinal walls and help move waste out more efficiently.

The Liver

The liver is your second largest organ. Its function is to help with digestion by producing bile. The bile helps break down fats into smaller units, which makes them easier to metabolize. It also processes carbohydrates, lipids, and proteins and it aids in the detoxification of the blood. The liver also stores nutrients, vitamins, and minerals that assist in the production of vital proteins and it keeps our immune system strong.

This is just a brief overview of the myriad of tasks your liver fulfills on a daily basis. As you can see, it is pretty important! In sum, your liver takes on the task of "taking out the garbage" from your body. Therefore, it can easily become overloaded with toxins, and our part is to help keep it healthy. How? For starters we need to look at our diets. (Everything always comes back to diet!) We must aim to eliminate anything that can cause stress to our liver, including all processed foods, refined sugars, alcohol, and medications. (Be sure to consult with your physician before cutting back or eliminating any medications that you are taking.) Foods that you may want to add to your diet because they promote liver health include avocados, dandelion greens, asparagus, walnuts, organic spinach, grapefruit, raw tomatoes, carrots, garlic, Brussels sprouts, and kale.

My personal favorite liver cleanser is kale. I will warn you to be careful with this one however, as it can be pretty potent! I once decided to detox my liver by going on a short juice cleanse using kale as my main vegetable. I was juicing about 16 ounces of kale at a time and only adding an apple and lemon with it. Around the second day of this cleanse, I began to feel woozy and I suddenly had a fever, chills, and a pounding headache. I was convinced that I had gotten the flu. The next morning I woke up and realized that I didn't have the flu but I had practically overdosed on kale! Now sometimes these symptoms, along with diarrhea, can be a normal and even a good sign that an overly-toxic body is detoxing, and this part of the process should only last a few short days before you will begin to feel much better than before. I personally had overdone it with this particular kale cleanse. To prevent making my mistake, it is a good idea for you to mix up your main vegetables, for example, by adding romaine lettuce instead of kale to some of your juices.

I have learned to pay close attention to my liver by how I am feeling. If I begin to feel sluggish and tired, I know that it's time to give my liver some TLC. I have also been taught throughout my years of body building that when lifting weights or exercising, the toxins that are stored in your muscles get released into your liver, so that the more you exercise, the more important it is to make sure you are consuming a lot of those liver-cleansing fruits and veggies, and that you should even consider going on an extended liver detox from time to time. If we don't keep our livers healthy, they can cause a trickle-down effect on the rest of our organs. So when you are keeping your liver healthy, you are keeping the rest of your body healthy as well.

The Skin

When we hear the word "organ," many of us think only about the liver, heart, stomach, etc. Skin may not even come to mind. Well, surprise! Your skin is actually your largest organ and one of the most important ones that you have. It is what keeps everything in place and held together. Thankfully, this is a simple organ to detox. Water is your skin's best friend because it helps to keep it hydrated and healthy. This means making sure that your diet includes a lot of foods that are high in water content such as cucumbers and melons.

Sweating is also a key component to keeping your skin toxin-free. It is your body's own way of detoxing and eliminating toxins that have built up. Even ladies shouldn't be afraid to sweat! I highly recommend using an infrared sauna, which helps your skin by making you sweat, and is said to remove heavy metals, radioactive particles, and improve the oxygenation of the blood.

Skin brushing is also recommended to help your body detox. To get started, you should buy a skin brush, which you can find at any local health food store. Before you shower or bathe, begin brushing and stroking your skin starting at your feet and moving upward toward your heart. This movement helps drain the lymphatic fluid back into your heart. Avoid stroking away from your heart, lest it put extra pressure on the valves within your veins and lymph vessels, which can damage vessels and cause varicose veins. After you get out of the shower or bath, dry yourself off vigorously and massage your skin with pure plant oils.

Detox Water

As I have already mentioned, it is important to keep hydrated, and water is one of the best ways to help your body eliminate toxins. If you happen to get bored with drinking plain water, consider "detox water." Detox water is simple and easy to make. Simply pick your favorite citrus fruit (lemon, orange, grapefruit, etc.) and pair it with your favorite fruits. Popular detox drinks consist of combinations such as lemon with cucumber, mint or watermelon, and lime with raspberries. Chop the fruits and put them into a jar with water. Allow it to sit for 30 to 60 minutes, then drink it. This provides a creative, healthy, and tasty pick-me-up that allows you to hydrate while flushing your system of toxins. Detox water isn't harsh on the body, so you can incorporate it into your day-to-day life, giving your water a little extra boost of flavor. I always add lemon to my detox water because I believe that it helps stimulate my digestive tract to break down fats and bile. You can research different fruits, veggies, and even herbs to decide for yourself which you feel your body would most benefit from. For example, adding cucumber may help reduce inflammation as well as act as a natural pain reliever. Mint leaves help calm stomach muscles, and grapefruit helps flush fat.

Healthy Detox Products

As I have mentioned throughout this chapter, your diet plays an important role in keeping your body toxin-free. I always prefer and recommend detoxing the natural way, however there are times when I will use a recommended product to help my body in the process. When looking for a good product, always research first, and read labels! Aim for a plant-based product that is organic. These products are for 21- to 30-day detox systems.

Needless to say, whenever you go on a detox or cleanse, you want to be sure to finish as well as you started. You do not want to finish your detox only to go right back to eating contaminated and processed foods. This will not only be a shock your body, but it will sabotage your hard work toward wellness.[8]

Grounding

Instead of "grounding," some people call it "earthing." No, grounding's not what your parents did to you when you were caught sneaking out or not doing your chores. It is the process of aligning yourself with the electromagnetic field of the earth. You see, the earth is an electrically charged planet and we are bioelectrical beings living on it.

Some people believe that grounding is an energy infusion, which has many great and powerful benefits. The way they believe it works is that it can restore, as well as help stabilize the bio-electrical circuitry. Bioelectrical circuitry manages everything from your physiology to your organs, as well as harmonize your basic biological rhythms. It is believed to boost self-healing mechanisms, to help boost your body's ability to heal itself while reducing inflammation and pain, improve your sleep cycle, and even promote feelings of calmness.

Putting skepticism aside, we do know that we are naturally drawn to grounding. Children love running around barefoot, and we all love walking on the sand barefoot (which is said to be the best form of grounding). This is said to be because our bodies' electrical fields are being normalized and brought into harmony and balance by the earth's electromagnetic field, without our even realizing it.

I would go barefoot all the time if I had my way. I believe that grounding has helped me immensely with my travels especially when I go into a different time zone. I first experimented with this when I took a trip to Switzerland. I tend to get severe jet lag, and though I had heard about grounding, I had never really paid much attention to it. On this particular trip, I figured that it wouldn't hurt to try. So after arriving, I took my shoes off every day, and walked around in the grass outside our hotel. I was amazed at how well I felt compared to other long-distance trips. I did experience slight jet lag, but not nearly as much as I was accustomed to.

Some of you may be skeptical of grounding, which is fine. I always tell people to seek things out for themselves before adopting anything as their own. I would recommend visiting the link in the endnote to read about how grounding can help alleviate various health conditions. In my opinion, this practice may be one of the best detox methods available to help achieve optimal health.

Fasting

Fasting has become more mainstream today than in the past, both for spiritual as well as health reasons. When people ask me what I think about fasting for weight loss or other health-related issues, I have to say that I don't believe one fast fits all. I always advise first and foremost to listen to your body.

Many years ago, Bill and I decided to go on an extended fast. I had fasted before, but not for more than a few days, so my body was not accustomed to what I put it through. I remember day 21 of our fast clearly: I was walking into the administration building at our church when I began to feel my body crashing—as if my brain and body had completely stopped working. There just happened to be a nurse in the office, and after she took one look at me she exclaimed, "What have you done to yourself?!" When I told her that I had been fasting, she immediately told me that I needed to eat right away, and grabbed some broccoli and white rice for me to eat. Let me tell you, that white rice and broccoli tasted like heaven in a bowl. What I took away from that experience is that I personally cannot do a juice or water fast; I have to feed my body food. Now if I fast, I follow a "Daniel fast," which eliminates all food except fruit, vegetables, and water.

As fasting has become more mainstream, there are now a variety of different ones to choose from. Here are a few types of fasts that I have seen people finish successfully. They may help promote weight loss as well as give your body a total detox.

Juice cleanse

Juice cleanses have probably become the most popular type of fast. Juicing raw fruit and vegetables is thought to allow the vitamins, minerals, and enzymes enter your bloodstream faster than if you were to eat them.[9] It is always recommended to juice more green vegetables than fruit because the sugars in the fruit can spike your blood sugar levels. I have seen people who have juiced primarily fruit become dependent on the sugar, which led to sugar cravings and occasional overeating after their fast, which is, of course, a discouraging result after so much hard work.

Water fast

This is a more extreme type of fast; you can have only water and lots of it. There are claims that doing this helps your body detox fully by allowing it to rest.[10] This type of fast is not recommended for those who are new to fasting. If you do decide to do a water fast, be sure to drink only good, filtered water that is free of contaminants.

Master cleanse

The master cleanse is another intense form of fasting. The idea behind it is to cleanse the colon of food and toxins. A solution made up of ten ounces of water, two tablespoons of lemon juice, two tablespoons of honey or maple syrup for calories, and 1/10 teaspoon of cayenne pepper is drunk between six and twelve times daily. Some people intensify the effects by incorporating a laxative tea twice a day, morning and night. A master cleanse can last anywhere from one to fourteen days, but you should always be under the supervision of a doctor, especially for a longer fast.

The Daniel fast

This cleanse is based on the story of Daniel in the Bible:

> *"Test your servants for ten days; let us be given vegetables to eat and water to drink. Then let our appearance and the appearance of the youths who eat the king's food be observed by you, and deal with your servants according to what you see fit." So he listened to them in this matter, and tested them for ten days. At the end of ten days it was seen that they were better in appearance and fatter in flesh than all the youths who ate the king's food.[11]*

The idea behind this is to follow the pattern of Daniel, and only eat fruits, vegetables, and water. Many people do this one for either spiritual or health reasons, and have found it valuable. As I mentioned, this is the type of fasting I do.

Note: Be sure to consult your physician before fasting, especially if you have a medical condition like diabetes. Also, don't undertake a fast if you're pregnant or nursing. Also note that detoxes are not a substitute for medical diagnoses or treatment.

I cannot stress enough my belief in the importance of keeping your body clean and detoxed. Whether you use foods to detox or good supplements, try to make this a part of your life. When you work at keeping your organs clean, your body will be an efficient well-working machine, and it will help your journey to health immensely.

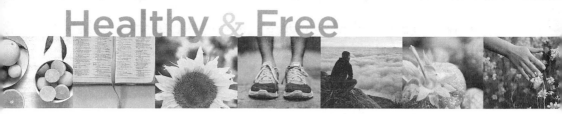

4.6

Nutritional Supplements

One of the things I love about the nature of God is His attention to detail. Nothing goes unnoticed by Him. I have seen this time and time again in my personal life as well as in the wonderful way that He designed the earth and the life cycles of all its creatures.

From the natural world down to the cells in our bodies, we see God's genius and brilliant handiwork. The same is true when you look at the wonderful way that He designed food to meet our bodies' needs. The vitamins and minerals found in our nutrition are essential to our ability to function properly. People often ask me if they need to take supplements as part of a healthy lifestyle. My answer is no— you probably don't need to *if* you are eating a diet full of nutrient-rich foods, staying hydrated, sleeping well, and have very little stress in your life. I am being humorous because we all know that the scenario I listed above is not the norm for most of us. Having said that, I really believe in the importance of drawing the majority of my nutrients from the whole, organic foods that I eat. So, I use supplements as an additional way to maintain a healthy lifestyle, which is especially important if you're as busy as I often am.

In this section I want introduce some supplements that I have found to help bring my body into optimal health. One thing that I have learned when searching for a good supplement is that it can get confusing when you find yourself faced with hundreds of different options. A good rule of thumb that I like to go by is to make sure that all my supplements are either fruit- or vegetable-based as well as certified organic, rather than synthetic vitamins. The word "synthetic" means "not of natural origins; prepared or made artificially." If you are using inexpensive "drugstore" vitamins, they are more than likely synthetic. Always read the labels, because your body deserves the very best.

A friend of mine is a colonics doctor, and part of her job is to analyze a person's waste in order to get an idea of their digestive health. She says that she can always tell which clients take synthetic vitamins, because their bodies cannot break them down, and they often pass through their systems completely whole. (This is why some people argue that if you use synthetic vitamins, you are flushing your money down the toilet.)

Now that you know which supplements to steer clear of, let's discuss which ones you should be taking. Please remember, before adding any supplements to your diet always speak to your healthcare provider.

Multivitamin

I recommend starting with a good, organic multivitamin. This will give you the recommended amount of vitamins and minerals for each day, which is beneficial especially for those who maintain busy lifestyles, exercise intensively, or are on low-calorie or vegan/vegetarian diets.

Omega-3s

Omegas-3 fatty acids are key to helping the body to reduce unhealthy inflammation, which is important because it is linked to a range of illnesses.[1] We get omega-3s from fish oils (like salmon), krill, flax seeds, chia seeds, and hemp seeds. Fish oils are the most common source for two types of omega-3 fatty acids (EPA and DHA[2]) and the oils from seeds are the best source of a third type of omega-3, ALA[3]; we need all three types. It is important to use good, organic fish oil (preferably from deep-sea fish).

Vitamin D

This vitamin is vital for your health because it helps your body to absorb important nutrients such as calcium and magnesium. Deficiencies in this vitamin can have severe consequences. Some of the symptoms of a vitamin D deficiency are dark skin under the eyes, feelings of depression, achy bones, digestive problems, and weight gain.

People can become deficient in this vitamin because they tend not to go outside enough, and if they do, they often smear strong chemical sunscreens onto their skin, which block their bodies' natural ability to create vitamin D from the sun. I found this out the hard way. Here I was doing everything that I knew to do to take care of my health by eating the right foods and exercising, yet no matter what I did, I could still tell that something was "off." I finally saw my naturopath, who ran some blood tests and found that I was extremely deficient in vitamin D; because of this, my body was unable to absorb all the nutrients that I was giving to it through my healthy diet.

Our bodies were designed to get vitamin D from sunshine and food (mostly animal-based).[4] Now I am not telling you to give up the use of sunscreen, but rather to be smart about when you use it. For instance, one of the best ways to get the benefits from the sun without damaging your skin is to go outside in the early morning. At that time of day the UV rays are not yet at their full capacity, so you can sit in the sun and allow your body to absorb vitamin D naturally for ten to fifteen minutes. Be sure that your legs, arms, and face are not covered, because those are the places where it is best absorbed. Doing this will also help balance out your melatonin levels, which will aid in maintaining healthy sleep patterns.

Probiotics

Probiotics promote good, healthy digestion, and overall health for your gut. Medications and antibiotics can destroy the good flora in your intestines, which, in turn, can cause digestive issues. After taking an antibiotic, it's a good idea follow up by taking a good probiotic to help replenish the flora that may have been destroyed. I feel that probiotics are a must for me so I take one religiously every day. Aside from taking a probiotic supplement, you can also get probiotics from foods such as organic yogurt, kefir, and kombucha. The latter is my favorite way to get good probiotics into my diet.

Enzymes

Enzymes keep us healthy and happy by breaking down the food we eat so that our bodies can absorb it and put its nutrients to use. In other words, they keep our metabolism healthy.[5] All living foods have enzymes in them, but when food is cooked the enzymes are drastically reduced and sometimes eliminated altogether. When enzymes are removed or reduced in our food, our bodies have a hard time with digestion. Enzymes are nature's 24/7 workforce—you could say that without them life is next to impossible.[6] I make sure that I am getting enough enzymes in my diet throughout the day either through the "living" food that I eat or in supplement form. I carry a bottle of enzymes in my purse with me and take them before every meal. A cooked steak, for example, is considered "dead food" due to its lack of enzymes, which makes it difficult to digest. So if you are grilling a T-bone for dinner, either have a salad or an enzyme supplement with it.

Because approximately half of our total enzyme production is used for digestion, some say that your body will pull reinforcements from other needed functions when there are not enough for digestion. Therefore, if your body is lacking in enzymes, your immune system can become weakened.[7] This is why I always recommend investing in a good, organic enzyme supplement to help support your body in its journey to wellness.

Home Remedies

I love finding good home remedies from the foods that we can normally find right in our kitchens. Here are some of my favorites, which have benefitted me the most on my journey toward a healthy lifestyle.

Turmeric

If you have turmeric buried somewhere in your spice cabinet to use for cooking, did you know that in addition to its ability to add wonderful flavor to specialty foods, it also carries many health benefits? Turmeric has been found to help fight cancer, relieve arthritis, control diabetes, reduce cholesterol levels, promote healthy immune and digestive systems, as well as aid in weight management. It may also help prevent Alzheimer's and liver disease.[8] Wow!

According to the Journal of the American Chemical Society, turmeric contains a wide range of antioxidant, antiviral, antibacterial, antifungal, anticarcinogenic, antimutagenic and anti-inflammatory properties. It is also loaded with many healthy nutrients such as protein, dietary fiber, niacin, vitamin C, vitamin E, vitamin K, sodium, potassium, calcium, copper, iron, magnesium and zinc.

Turmeric is fat-soluble. This means that it needs fat in order to dissolve. So, when taking turmeric, it's good to eat some good fat with it. If you are taking turmeric in a supplement form you can try to take your fish oil along with it or perhaps olive oil. That will help it absorb into your body and you will get the full benefit.[9] Some say that using ginger or black pepper with your turmeric can aid in the process of absorption.[10] I take a supplement that has ginger added to it.[11] It is safe to say that we can all benefit from this powerful spice in one way or the other, whether for cooking, sprinkling on foods, or even taken in a capsule form.

Apple Cider Vinegar

Apple Cider Vinegar (ACV) has been used for many years in kitchens throughout the world and is now becoming famous for its many health benefits. ACV is made from apples that have been fermented. Fermented foods are great for our health because they contain many enzymes, which, as I have said, help our bodies break down food and absorb the nutrients.

A friend of mine struggled with digestive problems. He didn't know what to do about it, so he went to God and asked Him. He sensed that He wanted him to add small amounts of apple cider vinegar to his diet, so he did, though he didn't know why. Because I know this friend well, I know that he had no idea how much ACV can help with digestive issues. What a great testimony! He trusted God's leading. I loved hearing about this story from him because it was a fresh reminder that God not only planned from the beginning of time to provide healing properties in the natural food we eat, but also that He is committed to lead us on this journey if we seek Him for advice. Remember to keep partnering with Jesus!

Among ACV's active ingredients are soluble fiber in the form of pectin, vitamin A, vitamin B_6, vitamin C, vitamin E, thiamin, riboflavin, niacin, pantothenic acid, beta-carotene, and lycopene. It also contains minerals such as sodium, phosphorus, potassium, calcium, iron, and magnesium. Some believe that ACV can actually change the way our digestive and circulatory systems work, in a positive way, making them more effective.[12]

When taking ACV, you can either take approximately one ounce straight (which, I will warn you, is tough for many people because it is so strong) or you can put an ounce of it in warm water and perhaps add some raw, local honey to help reduce the strong acidic taste. You should make sure that you are only using raw, unpasteurized, organic ACV with the "mother" left inside it. This looks like a stringy residue that is in the bottom of the jar and it is where the proteins, enzymes, and good bacteria can be found.[13]

Oil Pulling

Oil pulling is an ancient technique that has resurfaced in recent years due to its benefits for oral health. The way it works is to swish vegetable-based oil around in your mouth for 15 to 20 minutes. It is recommended to do this every morning; I do it a few times a week.

Here's how it works: **Step 1**: Put 1–2 teaspoons of oil in your mouth. I recommend organic coconut oil because it is antibacterial. Since coconut oil tends to set if it's cold, scoop it out as a solid and place it in your mouth. It should liquefy quickly. **Step 2**: Swish for 20 minutes. Yes, this may seem like a long time but this longer period is important. The oil needs time to be able to break through plaque and bacteria. I don't do this for more than 20 minutes however, because I don't want to risk retaining the bacteria that are being released. After a while you will notice that the oil is getting thicker and creamier, which is a good sign that it is working. **Step 3:** Spit the oil into a trashcan. Don't swallow it or spit the oil into the sink. **Step 4:** Rinse your mouth with warm water and then brush your teeth thoroughly. The water will help dissolve any oil that may be left over.[14]

Supplements for Travel

Over the many years that I have spent traveling, I learned the hard way how important it is to keep my immune and digestive systems in good working order. For years, I would suffer from jet lag, constipation, fatigue, and the general, unpleasant feeling of my body being off-kilter from changing time zones. I have learned some great tips along the way and I want to share with you some of the supplements I use when traveling.

- **Probiotics:** Finding a good probiotic has helped me more than I can put into words. I already covered probiotics earlier in this chapter. but I cannot stress enough the importance of keeping your gut healthy, especially when traveling. If you don't use one any other time, consider using it when you travel. You need them to help fight bugs or germs that you may come into contact with through local drinking water and food, especially when traveling to a developing nation.

- **Natural Calm:** Known as the "anti-stress drink," this product has saved me not only when I am traveling, but also when I am home.[15] It does two things for you. First, it contains magnesium, which helps you stay regular. (This is important. Let's just say that there is nothing like constipation to ruin a good trip.) Second, it is a good source of calcium, important for keeping muscles and bones healthy. I put the recommended dose in a glass of warm water right before I go to bed. On a side note, if you have a tendency to get constipated another great product to take is called Zypan by Standard Process. I have used it in the past and it works great for me.

- **Chlorophyll:** This is a wonderful healing product. It is known as a "super food" because it has many great benefits for your body, including strong antioxidants. It helps keep your cells healthy through eliminating free radicals and aids cleansing by eliminating toxic metals and carcinogens.[16]

- **Fiber:** I use food as my main source of healthy fiber, but you can find some good supplements as well. I always make sure that I have plenty of organic apples with me when I travel. In fact, if I am ever asked what I would like in my room, I always ask for organic apples. I buy packaged fruit leathers too, because they are easy to travel with, and they too contain lots of fiber.

- **Enzymes**: I went over the importance of enzymes earlier but I just cannot stress enough the importance of taking enzymes while traveling. They will help you digest your food and should be taken with every meal.

- **Melatonin**: This is a naturally occurring hormone that assists in managing our sleep and wake cycles.[17] I use this especially when traveling to help my body adjust to jet lag. Crossing time zones really messes with my sleep cycle and not being well rested on a trip can make any of us feel terrible. I take it at night right before I go to bed, in the dark. I recommend trying it at home before traveling just to be sure that it works for you. Also, never take more than the recommended dose. When I have taken too much melatonin, I have had really strange dreams.

With the exception of the melatonin, I use these travel supplements even when I am home.

Supplements for Athletes

I learned the hard way that when you exercise intensely, you must be sure to replenish your body with any nutrients that it may have lost and restore your electrolyte balance. It wasn't until I had some blood work done that I was told that I had depleted my body and I was dehydrated on a cellular level. Once I began taking supplements that a lot of other athletes take, I noticed that my body not only recovered but it also felt immensely better.

- **Omega-3 fatty acids (fish oil):** Fish oil is good for athletes because of its powerful anti-inflammatory properties.

- **B vitamins:** Vitamin B helps increase energy levels and neurotransmitter cofactors, so they can help improve mood and detox naturally, which is needed after exercise. The process of building and repairing muscle (processing protein) depletes B vitamins so if you're lifting heavy weights or damaging your muscle tissue in your work, you need to take extra B vitamins to help them rebuild.

- **Magnesium**: This is vitally important to athletes because it regulates heart rhythm, allows muscles to contract and relax properly, reduces blood pressure, and is necessary to activate the chemical compound ATP (adenosine triphosphate, important for energy transfer between cells).

- **Protein**: Protein is the muscle builder, so it is needed especially after lifting weights, which tears the muscle tissue, which then needs to be repaired. If protein is taken within ten minutes of a training session, it will reduce the amount of stress hormones (mainly cortisol) released as well.

- **Vitamin C:** During and after workouts are the optimal times to take vitamin C because it helps build collagen and repair muscle tissue. Trainers advise eating an orange right after a workout. Some advise that athletes should take a minimum of 4,000 to 8,000 milligrams a day and a maximum of 16,000 milligrams a day.

- **Coenzyme Q_{10} (CoQ_{10}):** Anyone who participates in strenuous training or is on statin drugs should take CoQ_{10}. The most usable form of CoQ_{10} for this purpose is ubiquinone (not to be confused with ubiquinol which enters the bloodstream and serves as an antioxidant but does not go into the cells to help with energy production). Many people take this supplement for their hearts, but this is a great one for recovery for athletes. Because it produces an increase in energy production, I do not recommend taking it at night.[18]

- **L-Glutamine:** Glutamine is important because it is the most abundant amino acid in the body[19] and it is found in over 61 percent of skeletal muscle.[20] Produced in the muscles, our bodies send it to the organs that need it the most. Because of this, glutamine levels can become depleted after strenuous physical activity, which then causes a decrease in energy levels, stamina, and recovery time. Glutamine helps the body metabolize fat and support new muscle growth. I normally take around 2000 milligrams a day in a capsule form. You can also take it as a powder.

- **Quercetin:** Quercetin is a strong antioxidant, anti-inflammatory, and antihistamine that is used for treating blood and heart conditions, high cholesterol, heart disease, and circulation problems. It has also been used to treat or prevent diabetes, cataracts, hay fever, peptic ulcers, schizophrenia, inflammation, asthma, gout, viral infections, chronic fatigue syndrome, cancer, and chronic infections of the prostate. Quercetin is used to increase endurance and improve athletic performance as well.[21] You can find it in foods such as kale, broccoli, and asparagus or you can take it in supplement form.

- **Turmeric with ginger:** This is one supplement that is used by many in the athletic field because inflammation is a real issue for bodybuilders and other athletes. These two herbs work well in reducing it. You can use your juicer and obtain them in natural form or take them as a supplement.

- **FitAid:** I recently discovered this drink at my gym and I have begun to use it in my daily life. You can use it both during and after you work out. The thing I like about this drink is that it is organic and contains glutamine, B complex, green tea extract, vitamins C, D, and E, glucosamine for joint health, amino acids/BCAAs, electrolytes for muscle stamina, CoQ_{10}, omega-3, turmeric, and quercetin. Because it contains most of the supplements mentioned above, it makes for a good recovery drink.

There are many other great supplements out there and you may need to shop around to find what works for you and what doesn't. Once again, before trying anything, always speak to your healthcare provider prior to use.

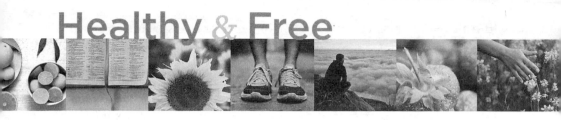

Healthy & Free

Chapter 5

Adrenal and Thyroid Health

But those who wait on the Lord
Shall renew their strength;
They shall mount up with wings like eagles,
They shall run and not be weary,
They shall walk and not faint.
—Isaiah 40:31, NKJV

Despite the title, this chapter is not only for those who have adrenal or thyroid gland problems. Instead, I want to touch on a subject that many of us are very familiar with—stress. Our culture has made our lives extremely demanding, and the glamorization of being busy hasn't made it any easier.

Not all stress is bad. Sometimes stress can be motivating, pushing us to achieve important goals. But it is vital to manage the stress in our lives rather than allowing the stress to manage us. First, I want to differentiate between the two main types of stress: acute stress, and chronic stress. Acute stress is more of your day-to-day short-term stress, like the stress of being caught in traffic, cooking dinner in a time crunch, hurrying to get to work on time, and so forth. Acute stress tends to come and go as the day goes on, and in most cases it's fairly simple to manage.

Chronic stress is the type we want to avoid. Doctors Lyle H. Miller and Alma Dell Smith describe chronic stress as the condition in which "a person never sees a way out of a miserable situation. It's the stress of unrelenting demands and pressures for seemingly interminable periods of time. With no hope, the individual gives up searching for solutions."[1] This kind of stress is extremely draining and potentially even fatal. Studies have shown that when you are under long-term, chronic stress, your body begins to think that it is being threatened, and in response it begins to shut down your major organs, including your nervous and immune system, endocrine system, and gastrointestinal system in order to preserve energy to fight off the attack against it. This, of course, can lead to sickness, memory loss, cancer, depression, insomnia, and a long list of other conditions.[2]

It is vitally important for our health that we learn how to manage chronic stress. In this chapter I am going to share with you part of my journey back to health. I want to show you how I recovered from the effects of chronic stress in my life.

My husband and I do a lot of traveling around the world for ministry. On average, I make about four or five international trips a year. Normally, they would be spread out throughout the year, which makes it easier on my body. However, in 2009, I reached a new record when by May my assistant and I had already made five international trips. My energy levels had dropped to such a low level that I looked at her and said, "I don't think I can do this anymore." Upon arriving home, I made an appointment with my doctor. After listening to my symptoms and running a saliva test, he diagnosed me with adrenal fatigue. Having never even heard of such a thing before, I began to ask a lot of questions. He finally looked at me and said, "Beni, if you were a mobile phone, I could charge you for an entire month and even then you wouldn't be fully charged." I felt the weight of his words.

I had been feeling overly tired, and doing the smallest tasks would take great effort. The long-distance traveling, speaking engagements, lack of good food, and poor sleep had finally caught up to me, and now I was paying the price. I was chronically stressed.

What do the adrenal glands have to do with fatigue? Well, the adrenals are small endocrine glands that sit right on top of our kidneys. They are responsible for helping our bodies respond to stress by releasing cortisol, a hormone that helps balance our response. A healthy adrenal gland will produce just the right amount of cortisol, while, an unhealthy adrenal will either produce too much cortisol or not enough. As with any other organ or muscle in our body, overworking the adrenal glands eventually leads to their under-functioning.

Allow me to paint a picture for you. You wake up in the morning, but despite pouring yourself a cup of coffee (or two), your day starts wearily. You don't actually "wake up" until around 10:00 A.M. Suddenly, you feel as though your coffee has finally begun to work and you experience a few hours of productivity, with some bursts of energy. You begin to plan the rest of your day, hoping that the energy will sustain itself, only to find yourself crashing again around 2:00 P.M. You sit at your desk as your eyes fight to stay awake. You drink another cup of coffee, but it seems to take every ounce of your energy just to walk to your car. You spend the next few hours in a blur as your concentration lessens, your mind feels foggy and the only thing appealing to you is your bed. You arrive home, vowing to make sure to go to bed early tonight, and begin cooking dinner. Then around 6:00 P.M., it seems as if your extreme exhaustion has lifted and suddenly you aren't in such a hurry to get to bed anymore. This cycle of exhaustion and bursts of energy continues to repeat itself; at 9:00 P.M. you feel exhausted, only to be re-energized around 11:00 P.M. Finally, although it was such a struggle to make it through the day, 1:00 A.M. rolls around, and you finally decide to go to bed.

Sound familiar to anyone? Symptoms of adrenal fatigue include:

- Daily cycles of energy bursts and fatigue

- Cravings for foods high in sugar and fat

- An increase in PMS and symptoms of menopause

- Mild depression

- Lack of energy

- Decreased ability to handle stress

- Muscular weakness

- Inflamed allergies

- Lightheadedness, especially when moving from a sitting to a standing position

- Decreased sex drive

- Frequent sighing

- Inability to handle foods that are high in potassium without combining them with fats and proteins

I was suffering from an overload of chronic stress. My body was trying to communicate to me; it was pleading for me to slow down. I had gotten to a point where just checking my emails overwhelmed me. I thank God that I had my assistant, because she was able to help shoulder the load when I was unable to.

I had to do a complete makeover of my life and my schedule. The first step was clearing my calendar. As hard as it was, I had to begin saying no to speaking events in order to avoid adding even more stress to my system. I began to allow myself to come home from work and tell myself that it was OK to just get into my pajamas and lounge. I was used to being extremely busy, so this was a hard step for me to take. I knew that allowing myself to rest without guilt would be crucial to my recovery, so I also began to make sleep a priority. Those who support the adrenal fatigue theory say that you should always try to sleep until 9:00 A.M. I know that sounds laughable to people who are not able to sleep that late for valid reasons such as kids, jobs, and other commitments. Still, the idea is to try to get at least eight hours of good sleep a day, because sleep is so crucial to recovering from adrenal fatigue.

Have you ever heard the expression that laughter is the best medicine? Well, it's true! In a study done by researchers at Loma University, they found this to be the case. They divided people into two groups, and gave everyone a saliva test. They then had one group sit in silence for 20 minutes, and the other group was given funny videos to watch. At the end of the time, they tested their saliva again, and also their ability to remember. They found that the group that had watched funny videos had a 43 percent increase in their recall ability, and their cortisol level had dropped significantly. The group that had sat in silence had only a 20 percent increase in recall ability and their cortisol level only decreased a small amount.[3] Laughter is healing, and it activates the "happy hormones" in our brains—the endorphins. I took this to heart, and I began consciously to make the effort to laugh. I began watching good clean sitcoms like *I Love Lucy* and *The Andy Griffith Show* as well as funny movies.

I also began taking care of myself nutritionally and physically. Because the adrenal glands regulate not only our emotional and mental stress, but also the physical stress that comes from diet and exercise, it is important to keep exercise light, and diet clean when recovering from adrenal fatigue. Walking and stretching are both ideal ways to get exercise without causing a lot of stress to the body. Also I was sure to get enough good meat in my diet, especially organic, grass-finished beef. (Grass-finished means that there is no corn added to the cow's diet at the end of its life.)

Last but certainly not least, I made sure to worship. I know that worshiping aligns my spirit and soul with God. I also believe that it aligns my body with Heaven, because we are triune beings—body, mind, and spirit are all one. I have experienced firsthand how being in the presence of God has really enabled my body to heal. This makes me think of a friend who came to speak at a service being held at our church. Although very few people knew at the time, she was struggling with serious health issues. While she was speaking, it seemed that every few minutes she would pause briefly. I asked her after the service what she was doing and she showed me that she had what she called an "invisible clock."[4] A doctor in Europe had recommended it for his cancer patients. He would have them set it to vibrate every ten minutes, and every time it vibrated they would worship God. I thought this was a genius idea. We tend to get so caught up in the hustle and bustle of our lives that it's easy to forget to talk to God. This invisible clock reminds us to posture our heart in reverence to Him. I immediately purchased one, and began wearing it every day—and worshiping. After about three weeks, I woke up one morning, and the first thing I noticed was how good I felt. I realized that even though I hadn't been aware of it, I had been feeling slightly depressed. I don't mean the chronic depression that many people deal with, but the less serious kind that comes from being overworked and overtired. My daily, conscious effort to worship had brought my spirit and soul into alignment, and my body quickly followed.

I had to do all of these things for about a year before I really started to reap the benefits and feel better. A year may seem like a long time, but we have to be patient on this journey. Our modern, instant-satisfaction culture has trained us to desire fast results, but God created us to be creatures of process.

Adrenal Makeover

If you are dealing with adrenal fatigue, you need to know what to do. I realize that dealing with any type of illness can be overwhelming, so I put together some basic, practical tips that may not only help you recover, but also give you a better overall quality of life.

- **REST**: Resting is vital to your recovery. Try to sleep in until 9:00 A.M. whenever possible. If you work, try lying down on your ten-minute breaks to help your body relax.

- **Laugh**: Watch good, clean sitcoms and videos. Go to dinner with your friends who always make you laugh. Watch old home videos. Whatever makes you laugh, do it!

- **Exercise**: Walking and stretching are great ways to keep your body active, and exercise gets your endorphins pumping. Remember, endorphins are the happy hormones; they will help you recover both mentally and physically. Bear in mind though, that easy does it. You do not want to set yourself back by putting more strain on your adrenal glands.

- **Minimize stress**: Go through your calendar and weed out the appointments and tasks that are not truly necessary. Learn to say "no." This will not only help alleviate stress, but it could also prevent further sickness from overworking yourself.

- **Eliminate negative people**: You know the type— negative and emotionally draining to be around. Avoid them when you have nothing to give. Learn to set boundaries. This may be tricky at times, especially if you live with or are related to negative people. A great book to help you with this subject is *Keep Your Love On* by Danny Silk.

- **Eat regular meals**: Many of us are busy from the moment we open our eyes in the morning. It is easy to forget to eat breakfast, or lunch for that matter, and we run ourselves dry until around 2:00 P.M. when we finally crash. Don't do this! Eating small meals every two or three hours will help your body stay energized, and give it the nutrients it needs to heal properly.

- **Chew your food**: Your mother used to tell you as a child to make sure you chew your food thoroughly before you swallow and she was right! Chewing your food helps your digestion. When we don't chew our food, our bodies have to work harder to break it down—and remember that you are trying to help your body with the workload right now. Chew your food as much as 30 or even 50 times per mouthful.

- **Have fun every day!** It will help reduce your cortisol levels, and alleviate stress. Having fun doesn't have to be expensive. It's a simple as playing a game with your kids, going to a local concert, or cooking a meal with your family. Whatever you love to do, do it!

- **Eat smart**: Keep your blood sugar from spiking, and then crashing, by sticking to whole, unrefined carbs such as sweet potatoes or quinoa, and always eat them together with a protein and a fat such as coconut or avocado oil. Avoid consuming junk food at all costs. I know from experience how easy it can be when you aren't feeling well to tuck yourself into bed with a box of donuts or a chocolate bar, but doing so will only make you feel worse and prolong your recovery. A large green juice may not seem as appetizing at first, but trust me when I say that your body will thank you.

- **Eat your veggies!** Once again, your mother was right—you need your vegetable to be healthy! Make sure that you are eating at least five or six servings of vegetables a day. They are loaded with vitamins and minerals that your body needs to heal. Experiment and explore until you find vegetables that you like better than the basic frozen peas and mushy broccoli that many of us grew up on.

- **Use your salt shaker**: Yes, you read that correctly. I am advocating salt. Many of us are used to hearing that sodium is bad for us, but I am here to say that I disagree. The normal table salt that we find in our stores and homes is not good for us because it's been bleached, processed, and stripped of all its good nutrients. However, our bodies desperately need the trace minerals that are contained in salt in its pure form. Many of us crave salty foods because our bodies are starving for the trace minerals found in the right kind of salt. I personally recommend Pink Himalayan salt and Celtic sea salt.

- **Vitamin C**: Vitamin C aids in replenishing and healing the adrenal glands by providing important antioxidants. Add as much as 2,000–5,000 milligrams a day to your diet.

- **Calcium and magnesium**: Calcium helps calm your nervous system while magnesium helps manage your blood pressure. Both are directly related to keeping your cortisol, the "stress hormone," low.

- **Vitamin B complex**: Vitamin B is essential in helping you increase your energy level. It's a good replacement for caffeine and other stimulants, because it's a natural vitamin that your body needs. Make sure that you are using one that is high in B_6 and pantothenic acid.

- **Vitamin E**: Vitamin E helps promote a healthy immune system, and when your immune system is healthy, your chances of getting sick are decreased, resulting in less stress on your body and adrenals. Try finding a vitamin E that has tocopherols, to help your body better absorb the vitamin.

- **Licorice root**: Now, I'm not suggesting you drop everything, run to your local grocery store, and buy a package of licorice candy. That is far from the pure form of the licorice plant that gave this treat its name. Licorice root promotes a healthy digestive system and healthy cholesterol levels, and it also may help heal the liver.[5]

As always, please consult with your healthcare provider before adding any supplements to your diet. Remember that being in good communication with both your doctor and your body is key to making lasting changes. Now that we've covered the basics in adrenal health, I want to move onto a closely related topic, the thyroid gland.

The Importance of Thyroid Health

The importance of the thyroid gland to your overall health and well-being has become a popular subject today. I didn't hear much about it growing up, but having battled thyroid sickness myself, I now know how important it is to consider this gland's health. A staggering 20 million Americans struggle with thyroid issues, and 80 percent of them are completely unaware of their condition![6]

I have counseled and spoken to many people who feel defeated, because despite their best efforts to lose weight, they seem to be stuck, no matter how restrictive their diet may be or how intensely they work out. Because of my experience, I now know to advise them to make sure to get their thyroid checked.

Before we go any further, what is the thyroid? It is one of the eight major glands in your body and it is responsible for the production of hormones that control your metabolism, growth, mood, development, and body temperature. When the thyroid becomes weak, the entire body is affected. Symptoms of a thyroid condition include decreased energy, depression, reduced heart rate, dry skin, weight gain, hair loss, constipation, and the inability to feel warm. (It's easy to miss some of the symptoms for a thyroid condition because many of us are used to feeling overworked, overstressed, and undernourished.)

If you can relate to these symptoms, I recommend seeing your doctor. However, it's important that you go in knowing exactly which tests you want done. Many doctors typically do not run a full thyroid test and will only test your pituitary gland, which is a gland that controls the thyroid. It's an important test, but it does not give you a full enough picture of how healthy your thyroid is. When you go to your doctor, specifically ask to have them run the T4, T3, and rT3 hormone tests. Having these results will give you a full picture of your thyroid health.

A simpler way to test it is by taking an iodine test. Bear in mind, this is not a complete and accurate thyroid test, but it may tell you whether your body is low in iodine or not. Since iodine deficiency is linked to thyroid sickness this test may help shed some light on whether your thyroid is healthy or not. Simply purchase some red-colored iodine from any local drugstore, apply a patch to the inner part of your wrist and let it dry. If your iodine levels are healthy, the red stain should remain visible for 24 hours. My naturopath performed this test on me, and within 30 minutes the iodine had completely disappeared from my skin! It was a pretty good indicator that my thyroid might be in bad shape, and in need of some intervention.

I like to call the T3 hormone a dream come true because it helps regulate your body back to happiness by warming you up, lifting your mood, increasing your energy, and even helping make your hair grow. There are ways to naturally increase the production of T3 by adding some good vitamins and minerals to your diet, such as iodine, selenium, iron, zinc, vitamins A, riboflavin (B_2), B_{12}, and B_6. I will discuss where these can be found later in the resource section. The other hormone, rT3, acts as a balancing hormone and helps flush any excessive T4 that may be in your system.[7] Because of that, you need to be extremely careful to keep your rT3 levels balanced because excessive amounts of rT3 will cause too much T4 to be pushed out of your system, and also lead to feelings of fatigue and depression.

As if we need another reminder about the importance of learning to manage stress, stress is known to be a large factor among other factors that contributes to high or abnormal rT3 levels. Some of the other factors include vitamin D and iron deficiency, estrogen dominance, and high TPO antibodies (TPO is an enzyme found also in the thyroid).

Various elements called halogens make an impact on the thyroid gland, some good (such as iodine) and some not so good (such as fluorine, chlorine, and bromine), which displace the needed iodine. To keep your thyroid healthy and able to produce the hormones that are vitally needed to support your body, alternative practitioners suggest that you steer away from ingesting fluorine, chlorine, and bromine, bearing in mind that they are common in our tap water, swimming pool water, and disinfectants.

Thyroid Makeover

Let's say you can relate to the symptoms that points toward a thyroid problem. You've been to your doctor, you've taken your iodine test, and it is now painfully clear that your thyroid is in dire need of some TLC. What do you do next? Well, you have a few options, and it's important that you try to stay in tune with what your body is telling you. Doing a thyroid makeover will not only help get your thyroid back on track, but will also rejuvenate your entire body.

Let's first start with some simple tools to adjust your diet. Hippocrates is often quoted as having said, "Let food be thy medicine and medicine thy food." Making positive changes to your diet can help your thyroid immensely. First, consider reducing your carb intake. Grains and gluten are the thyroid's greatest enemies since they can cause inflammation. This is why many people have found great success by keeping to a paleo diet. Also make sure that you are eating protein with every meal because protein will help keep your energy levels up. A lack of protein in your diet may cause you to feel fatigued.[8] Next, eliminate or reduce your caffeine intake. Yes, that will probably include saying goodbye to your beloved daily latte, but you will thank yourself later. Caffeine can wreak havoc on your thyroid. I've found some good alternatives to caffeine such as herbal teas like Yerba Matte and Tulse. Another option is to make a juice of carrot, kale, apple, and turmeric, which will give your body a natural and healthy energy boost.

Another essential part of your thyroid makeover is to rest. This is easier for some than others, along with eliminating stress. Yet learning to manage and "get away" from your stress will help pave the road back to health. When I need a break from a stressful situation, I have been known to escape into a dark or dimly lit room. Try playing some worship music or something that will help your mind to relax. You can practice deep breathing and meditating on Scriptures. Massages are recommended to help lower cortisol levels. Go for a walk or take a hot bath. Do whatever you find relaxing and peaceful.

Some key vitamins and minerals that are believed to promote healthy thyroid function can be added through your diet or by taking (good organic) supplements.

- **Iodine**: Iodine is needed by the thyroid for hormone production. Iodine is found in seaweed or sea vegetables, cod, dairy, eggs, potatoes, and grains. I went on an iodine supplement for two months myself (from the company Standard Process).[9] However, it is possible to take too much iodine, so please be sure to keep checking your levels with your healthcare provider to prevent any complications.

- **Selenium**: This mineral helps bind the iodine in the thyroid, making it harder for other halogens to dislodge and replace it. Selenium can be found in Brazil nuts, cashew nuts, some fish such as yellow tuna, halibut, turkey, chicken, lentils, oatmeal, and bananas.

- **Vitamin D**: A lack of vitamin D has been linked to thyroid sickness, and adding this into your diet will help combat fatigue. The best way for your body to get vitamin D is to get some sun, since vitamin D is produced whenever the skin (and eyes) are exposed to direct sunlight. If you don't get enough sunshine, or you live in a place where the climate doesn't cooperate with your need for natural vitamin D production, you can get it through eating foods such as fatty fish (like salmon, trout, and sardines), as well as beef liver, egg yolk, dairy, and mushrooms (if they have been exposed to UV light).

- **Vitamin B_{12}**: Vitamin B_{12} deficiency has also been linked to thyroid sickness. Vitamin B_{12} will also help give energy levels a boost. This vitamin is found in poultry, fish, eggs, dairy, and organic supplements.

- **Probiotics and enzymes**: Probiotics and enzymes may not only benefit the thyroid but the entire body; they play a pivotal role in keeping the gut healthy. Many health food stores carry quality organic probiotic supplements. Another good source is kombucha, the fermented tea.

- **Ashwagandha**: This Indian root is known for its rejuvenating and energy-boosting effects as well as its ability to protect the digestive system and improve memory.

- **Essential oils:** There are many essential oils that may help support your thyroid. When I was recovering from thyroid sickness, I applied two drops of myrtle oil to my thyroid area three times a day. The company Young Living makes a capsule called Thyromin that is specifically designed to help rejuvenate and support the thyroid.

Many healthcare providers are willing to prescribe thyroid medications to their patients. Only you can decide if that is the right course of treatment for you. If you decide to take thyroid medication, you may be able to take a thyroid supplement as well. Just make sure that you do not take them at the same time. (For example, if you take your medication in the morning, take your supplement at night.) As always, make sure you consult your doctor before adding any supplements to your diet.

I know that we just covered a large amount of information which might feel overwhelming. Remember, as I have said before, this is a journey, not a race. Give yourself time. Live one day at a time, and be generous when it comes to giving yourself grace in the process. God will be faithful to meet you where you are, and help guide you along the way.

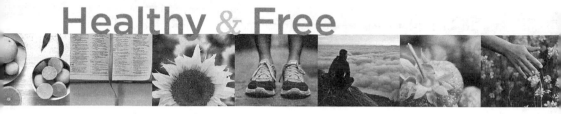

Chapter 6

Essential Oils

Note: Always consult with your doctor before using any supplements or oils. I am only sharing with you what has worked for me, and am neither advising nor promoting the use of oils in place of medication. Please use caution when using them.

Just a few years ago, it seemed as though hardly anybody knew much about essential oils, nor did they use them for their health. Now, everywhere I go people are talking about the benefits of their medicinal properties. At the same time, people who don't understand how essential oils work seem to be afraid of them, even labeling them as a New Age practice. Personally, I had been using essential oils on and off for a number of years, but hadn't gone to the effort of studying them until relatively recently. The more that I began investigating them, the more that I realized they could play an important role in my healthy lifestyle—especially when I discovered just how often the Bible refers to the healing properties of oils. There are actually a total of 670 references to oils in the Bible.[1]

In biblical times, modern pharmaceutical medicine did not yet exist, so medical providers sought out natural methods. For example, the priests were commanded by God to use a particular mixture of oils to perform a temple cleansing:

> Then the Lord said to Moses, "Take the following fine spices: 500 shekels of liquid myrrh, half as much (that is, 250 shekels) of fragrant cinnamon, 250 shekels of fragrant calamus, 500 shekels of cassia—all according to the sanctuary shekel—and a hin of olive oil. Make these into a sacred anointing oil, a fragrant blend, the work of a perfumer. It will be the sacred anointing oil. Then use it to anoint the tent of meeting, the ark of the covenant law, the table and all its articles, the lampstand and its accessories, the altar of incense, the altar of burnt offering and all its utensils, and the basin with its stand. You shall consecrate them so they will be most holy, and whatever touches them will be holy. Anoint Aaron and his sons and consecrate them so they may serve me as priests. Say to the Israelites, **'This is to be my sacred anointing oil for the generations to come'**" (Exod. 30:22–31, NIV).

God had Moses create a very specific oil blend. The particular oils used in this Scripture are associated with healing and emotional peace, which then became part of the properties of the sacred anointing oil. I find it interesting that this sacred oil blend was originally restricted for the exclusive use of the Old Testament priests. In the New Testament Peter tells us that God has now called us *all* His royal priesthood and His people (see 1 Pet. 2:9). What used to be limited to the Levites for priestly ministry is now accessible to all of us. In the context of spiritual as well as physical health, I find it intriguing that the priests of the Old Testament were often sought out to treat medical conditions. This supports my understanding of helping people live healthy lives as a divine mandate to us as New Testament believers.

An example of the Old Testament application of essential oils in ceremonial settings is found in the book of Leviticus.

> *The Lord said to Moses, "These are the regulations for any diseased person at the time of their ceremonial cleansing, when they are brought to the priest: The priest is to go outside the camp and examine them. If they have been healed of their defiling skin disease, the priest shall order that two live clean birds and some **cedar wood**, scarlet yarn and **hyssop** be brought for the person to be cleansed. Then the priest shall order that one of the birds be killed over fresh water in a clay pot. He is then to take the live bird and dip it, **together with the cedar wood, the scarlet yarn and the hyssop, into the blood of the bird that was killed over the fresh water. Seven times he shall sprinkle the one to be cleansed of the defiling disease, and then pronounce them clean**"* (Lev. 14:1–7, NIV).

In his book, *The Healing Oils of the Bible,* David Stewart states, "They [the priests] were all apothecaries and perfumers who mixed the various oils and herbs for anointing, for incense, and for healing. They also cared for the temple buildings and grounds, keeping them clean, attractive and in good repair."[2] As I read this I began to wonder, "Since we are all now considered God's holy priests, what temple does the Lord give to us to care for? What does this look like for us today?" The answer lies in what Paul wrote: "Do you not know that your bodies are temples of the Holy Spirit, who is in you, whom you have received from God? You are not your own" (1 Cor. 6:19, NIV). While we no longer have temple buildings to care for and cleanse, we've been given a much greater and more valuable temple that can be anointed with oil and used by God.

Here are some more biblical examples of the use of oils for medicinal as well as spiritual uses, and even for cosmetic treatments:

> *Before a young woman's turn came to go in to King Xerxes, she had to complete twelve months of beauty treatments*

prescribed for the women, six months with oil of myrrh and six with perfumes and cosmetics (Esther 2:12, NIV).

And they cast out many devils, and anointed with oil many that were sick, and healed them (Mark 6:13, NKJV).

Then Mary took a pound of very costly oil of spikenard, anointed the feet of Jesus, and wiped His feet with her hair. And the house was filled with the fragrance of the oil (John 12:3, NKJV).

Purge me with hyssop, and I shall be clean; wash me, and I shall be whiter than snow (Ps. 51:7 NKJV).

*The priest is to take some **cedar wood, hyssop** and scarlet wool and throw them onto the burning heifer.... Then a man who is ceremonially clean is to take some **hyssop,** dip it in the water and sprinkle the tent and all the furnishings and the people who were there. He must also sprinkle anyone who has touched a human bone or a grave or anyone who has been killed or anyone who has died a natural death* (Num. 19:6,18, NIV).

Now that we have seen how oils play a vital part in the Bible, let's take a look at how they work from a scientific standpoint. I want to explain why essential oils are effective and powerful alternative tools in healing our bodies and minds. God gave us five senses: sight, smell, hearing, taste, and touch. Out of these, smell is the only sense that activates the limbic lobe of the brain, which is often referred to as the emotional control center.[3] Emotions ranging from fear, joy, nostalgia, anxiety, to depression are controlled by the limbic lobe. When you smell lavender, for example, which is known for its calming and balancing effects, the scent molecules travel into your nose and get trapped by olfactory membranes, which stimulate the olfactory bulb in the brain, where information about the scent molecules and their effect are processed. The olfactory bulb then sends its processed information to the gustatory center and limbic system. The gustatory and limbic system are both control centers in the brain responsible for physical and emotional well-being, affecting functions such as the heart, blood, memory retention, and hormones. Once the lavender scent molecules have reached this point, your brain begins to send messages to your limbic lobe (again, the place where emotions are controlled) and other organs in your body, stimulating them to relax. In other words, a lavender essential oils' powerful scent has a direct and tangible impact on how peaceful, healthy, and happy you feel. Other essential oils help to stimulate an increase in oxygen to the brain, which also helps balance emotions, increase energy levels, and prevent memory loss. Imagine the change you'd experience in your quality of life if you felt emotionally balanced and had enough energy to get through the day!

Peppermint oil is my "go-to" oil because of its vast benefits and healing properties. Dr. Alan Hirsch conducted a study in which he used peppermint oil to stimulate weight loss in dieters who had previously been unsuccessful in their attempts at weight loss. Over the course of the six-month study, the results were outstanding, as the average weight loss was about 30 pounds per participant.[4] This is because the scent molecules in peppermint stimulate the part of the brain that controls feelings of satiety and fullness. Aside from helping with weight loss, peppermint has also been reported to help relieve and reduce headaches, muscle tension, digestive issues, and inflammation in the body.

A dear friend of mine, Christa Black Gifford, was once a skeptic of essential oils before experiencing their potential for healing for herself. I love the beautiful testimony from her blog:

> I was a bit skeptical when my mom wanted to rub me down with oils for the nasty case of bronchitis that had come to knock me off my feet. I looked a bit like a pathetic mummy after she rubbed Young Living Thieves Oil (cut with a carrier oil) all over my chest and throat every hour upon the hour, then wrapping me up with a scorching hot towel. Her diffuser poured billowing steam laced with something

called Thieves and R.C. into my nostrils, and she kept coming by to reapply a few drops to the soles of my feet. If I'd had enough energy to actually care, I would have protested. But because I felt like a cat had crawled inside my body and scratched up my throat, I would have let her do just about anything if it brought some relief. You know how you just know your body? The icky sick that I felt growing inside of my throat and lungs that day was the same sickness that I had felt many times before—and it had always resulted in a week in bed. But the next morning the strangest thing happened—I woke up almost completely well.[5]

The following is a testimony about essential oils from another friend of mine who struggled with insomnia for as long as she could remember, and had great success using essential oils.

At the age of 11, I began taking melatonin and by the time I was 19, my insomnia got so bad that I began taking Ambien, Klonopin, and Trazodone, among many other types of sleeping medications. I had been on a rollercoaster when it came to my sleep, and I felt hopeless thinking that I could never have a normal sleep life. Not too long ago, I discovered essential oils, and I began toying with the idea of coming off of my sleeping meds and using just the oils. I began using two drops of lavender, and two drops of cedarwood, and would rub them on the bottom of my feet. I was amazed because within one week, I began sleeping better than I have ever slept before! I am so thankful that I can now have a normal sleep life without the use of prescription drugs.

If you are new to the world of essential oils, the wide range to choose from can seem overwhelming. My advice is to start with some basic oils and learn which ones work the best for you. Here a few of my personal favorites that I have found to be beneficial when I used them consistently.

- **Cedarwood, Xlang Xlang and lavender oils:** For those who struggle with insomnia or have trouble unwinding, these oils have relaxing and calming properties, which may help. I place a couple of drops of each on my hands, rub them together and apply the oil to my left toe and upper foot area. You may be thinking, "Why the toes?" Experts say it's because the skin of your toes is the most porous on your body, which allows the oil to enter your system faster.

- **Peace and Calming Blend (from Young Living):** Just as its name states, this blend of essential oils may enhance a sense of peace, and promises to have a calming effect on your mind. If I know that I am going to have a busy or somewhat stressful day, I also will apply this to my left toe, the back of my neck, and finish off with a few deep inhalations, which I have found helps increase its calming effect on me.

- **Stress Away (Young Living roll-on):** Again, just as its name implies, this blend may help promote stress relief. I roll it on the back of my neck on extra-stressful days.

- **Idaho Blue Spruce:** I find this to be helpful for my mind when placed right on the hairline of my forehead. It relaxes both my mind and body and contains alpha-pinene acid and limonene, which serve as decongestants for mucous membranes.

- **Copaiba:** This oil has been used for its anti-inflammatory properties, and it may support healthy brain function. I place it just above my temples.

- **Idaho Balsam Fir:** This oil may help balance cortisol levels to help keep your body healthy and safe from the effects of stress. I apply this at the mid-shaft of my nose three to eight times a day.

- **Lemongrass:** This oil is said to have antifungal, antibacterial, antiparasitic, and anti-inflammatory properties. It may help promote lymphatic flow, and is recommended for purification and digestion. I add three drops to a capsule and take it as a pill.

- **Myrtle:** I like to think of this as a miracle oil because of its many different uses and benefits. It may help boost your immune system as well as provide support to your thyroid. Some also use it to help with concentration or sleep. I apply this oil in several different ways at the same time (typically in the morning). First, I put a drop on the tip of my tongue or the roof of my mouth. I also apply a few drops on my hands to stroke over the thyroid area of the throat. I then put my hands to my nose and take three deep breaths to inhale the full aroma.

I also like to use a couple of drops each of lemongrass, clary sage, lavender, and helichrysum oils on my feet both in the morning and the evening. I apply them to the liver points on my feet to help my liver detox.[6]

Some essential oils are safe for use with children. However, please use caution when doing so. Remember that their bodies are much smaller than ours, and normally do not need as strong a dosage. Young Living offers a collection of oils specifically made for children called KidScent Oil Collection. Some others that are safe to use are Lavender, Chamomile, and Gentle Baby by Young Living oils.

Note: As a final reminder, always use caution when applying oils. Make sure you research the ones you choose before using them on yourself or your family. Don't just use any oil you find, but make sure that it is 100 percent organic and pure.

Essential Oil Recipes

Nerve Damage

(May help restore damaged nerves, increase circulation, pain management, and infection protection. Apply 3–4 drops topically to the area of damage 2–3 times per day.)[7]

15 drops geranium

10 drops helichrysum

10 drops wintergreen

8 drops marjoram

6 drops cypress

5 drops peppermint

2 drops clove

2 drops lemon

Hemorrhoids

(May help relieve hemorrhoid discomfort. Combine the following, and apply to affected area 2–3 times daily)[8]

10 drops carrier oil

3 drops chamomile

4 drops lavender

5 drops geranium

Joint Pain

(May help relieve joint pain and discomfort. Mix ingredients together and apply topically as needed.)[9]

4 drops juniper

3 drops peppermint

3 drops marjoram

3 drops Roman chamomile

3 drops helichrysum

3 drops ginger

1 teaspoon coconut oil

Hypothyroid

(May help lessen hypothyroid symptoms. Combine ingredients, and apply to thyroid area and bottoms of your feet three times daily.)[10]

10 drops clove

10 drops myrrh

8 drops frankincense

8 drops lemongrass

2 tablespoon fractionated coconut oil

Digestion/Constipation

(May help relieve digestion or constipation symptoms. Combine ingredients and massage onto the belly in a clockwise circular motion 2–3 times daily.)[11]

5 drops coriander

7 drops orange

4 drops lemon

2 drops ginger

4 drops peppermint

4 ounces fractionated coconut oil

Insomnia

(May help relieve insomnia. Whip the coconut oil until it has a creamy consistency. Combine ingredients to make a soothing lotion, and apply at bedtime as needed.)

8 drops lavender

8 drops valerian

8 drops Young Living Peace and Calming Blend

¾ cup coconut oil

Migraines

(May help relieve migraines. Combine ingredients and apply around the crown of your head and forehead.)

2 drops marjoram

2 drops geranium

2 drops helichrysum

1 drop lavender

2 drop peppermint

2 frankincense

2–4 tablespoons coconut oil

For migraine relief, you can also apply one drop of peppermint oil to your hands and cup them around your nose. Take five deep, slow breaths, and then apply one drop of peppermint oil on your forehead and one drop on three different places on your scalp.

Young Living also has a great blend specifically designed for migraine relief called M-Grain. It contains marjoram, peppermint, lavender, basil, Roman chamomile, and helichrysum, which can be applied topically.

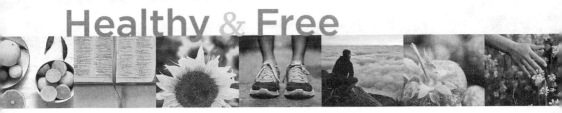

Healthy & Free

Chapter 7

The Skinny Obsession

Those who look to him are radiant, and
their faces shall never be ashamed.

—PSALM 34:5, ESV

I would like to introduce to you Rihanna Teixeira. When she became my intern to help me write *Healthy and Free*, I was not initially aware of the load she was carrying on her life. As I listened to her journey of recovery from bulimia, I knew that I had to put her story in this book.

Eating disorders affect approximately 24 million people in the United States alone, and sadly, that number seems to be increasing.[1] Rihanna's story gives a glimpse of what it is like when the normal desire to be thin becomes unhealthy and dangerous. I am certain that many people will find hope and healing through her story.

It didn't start as a disorder. It didn't start as a disease. A sixth-grader has no way of comprehending how the seemingly harmless act of skipping breakfast would begin a 14-year journey that would result in her fighting for her life. I was that sixth-grader, and I just wanted to lose a little bit of weight. All the other girls I knew, both peers and adults, seemed to want the same thing. Around that age, a girl's body begins to change and takes on a curve and shape that are quite different from the rail-thin body that she has known all her life.

In addition to the physical changes that take place at that time in a girl's development, life happens. Tragic and traumatic events are no respecter of persons or age, and as I look back I can see that my mind and heart didn't know how to process all the physical and emotional loss of family that I was experiencing. I learned early on that life was scary. At any moment someone I loved could be taken away from me, either through natural causes or because they had decided to find another family—other people to love besides us.

Hunger took that pain away. The ache in my stomach distracted me from the pain in my heart. I could control my hunger pangs, which in a funny way made me feel powerful when I couldn't control the emotional pain that I was feeling.

As I said, skipping breakfast seemed harmless to me. Most adults did it, and my friends told me it would help prevent me from gaining weight. I don't remember if it was effective or not because I was only 12 years old. To tell the truth, I didn't have weight to lose. However, I tend to be an all-or-nothing type of person, so I figured that if cutting breakfast out of my diet would help me lose weight, surely skipping lunch would as well. I spent the next few years in a perpetual state of hunger and self-defeat as I began associating food with guilt. My mind was dwelling on food all the time. I was consumed with cravings, daydreams of foods high in sugar and fat, and an obsessive need to watch people eat what I wouldn't allow myself to have.

This went on for a few years until I was a sophomore in high school. I remember the day as if it were yesterday. I was driving home from school and made a beeline for the kitchen as soon as I stepped foot in the door. I ate everything I could get my hands on. Boxes of cereal were gone within minutes, a dozen granola bar wrappers hidden in the trash, cartons of ice cream, peanut butter by the spoonful and other food leftovers—all consumed in a frenzy. I had never binged prior to that day, and to be honest, I had never heard of it before. I lay in my bed as shame began to weigh heavily on me. Over and over again I recounted every calorie I had eaten. I was desperate to get rid of the food in my stomach, but I didn't know how.

As I look back on that day, I can see that it was a turning point for me, after which I began to go down an even darker road. I had become so disconnected from my heart that as it began screaming louder and louder, I had to find a way to drown it out more forcefully. In hindsight, I see it as the day I allowed bulimia to take a root in my heart. I felt too ashamed to ask for help because I didn't understand what had happened, but I just knew it was wrong.

Life carried on, and I continued to pursue the dreams that I had had since childhood. When I was five years old, I had gotten my hands on one of my mom's Amy Grant records. I still remember dancing in the living room to her music, and dreaming of the day when I would be the next Amy Grant. From that point on, my life revolved around voice lessons, choir practices, music performances, and traveling. Now that I was about to graduate from high school, very little had changed. My parents traveled with me back and forth to various music competitions and vocal instructors as I tried to make it in the music industry. That industry is brutal no matter who you are, but add low self-esteem and an eating disorder to the mix and it is a recipe for disaster. My weight began to go up and down as I continued to battle bulimia. I seemingly ate a perfect diet and was often praised for my willpower, but in secret I would cram as many calories as I could while being sure to get rid of them any way I knew how. It goes without saying that being a singer, vocal and throat health are of the utmost importance. Knowing that I was abusing the only thing that I truly valued, my voice, only added more shame and guilt.

Finally, around the age of 19, my parents and close friends began to take notice and worry. They became aware that my "health" obsession went to a level that sucked every ounce of joy and energy out of me. My nights were spent bingeing and purging in secret, and my days would begin with puffy eyes and a disconnected heart. Eventually, my parents knew that they had to do something to intervene, and I soon found myself in an inpatient treatment facility in the middle of Arizona for four months.

I wish that I could say that after four months of treatment, I found freedom, and that the rest is history, but that wouldn't be true. For me, I came out worse than when I went in. Having spent so much time with girls who battled the same demons that I did, I learned new tricks and secrets regarding how to successfully master and mask an eating disorder. After treatment I found myself in the party scene, which I had sworn to myself I would never get into. Night after night I tried to fill a place in my heart that only knew emptiness. I would spend my days obsessing over calories, food, and exercise, and I would spend my nights as the life of the party, taking shot after shot, only to find myself alone in the bathroom bingeing on foods I wouldn't dare touch sober, and purging at the end of the night.

This was what the next four years of my life looked like. I used bulimia to keep me safe from the people around me who hurt me. In my broken emotional logic, family, friends, and ex-boyfriends couldn't hurt me if I was already hurting myself. Their rejection couldn't get to me because I had already rejected myself. Day after day, binge after binge, I kept myself from thinking about what they did to me by thinking incessantly about food. Thoughts of what I could and couldn't have, how I should exercise, and how I should look consumed every part of me, to the point that my dreams didn't even matter to me anymore. All I wanted was to be skinny. Every morning started off in a battle in which I would try to give myself pep talks to convince myself that today would be the day when I would get better, that today would be the day I would eat a perfect diet like a normal person. No matter how much I hoped, it was never "that day."

Around the age of 24, I had a radical encounter with God. I was alone in my bedroom, having just finished bingeing and purging. I was lying on my bed with my head spinning from my self-abuse, not to mention that I was still recovering from a night of heavy partying. I looked on my nightstand, and there lay a Bible that someone had given me years before. I had never opened it, but I was desperate, and something within me said that what I needed was mine for the taking inside that book. I opened it randomly, and the page fell to Psalm 18:24, which reads, "God rewrote the text of my life when I opened the book of my heart to His eyes."[2] I immediately began sobbing as I realized that even though I had spent my entire life escaping from own heart, I could never fully escape the reach of God. God's sweet presence filled my room, and I knew that I was being given a second chance at life.

After that night I slowly began to withdraw from the party scene, and I found myself at every church service I could attend. A hunger for God that I had never known could exist had been opened inside of me. I wish that I could say that I was delivered from bulimia then, but I wasn't. Now that I had given up drinking and partying, my bulimia actually seemed to take a turn for the worse. I carried a lot of shame because I felt that since I was going to church and pursuing God that I should be free. I spent many nights crying out on my bathroom floor to God, pleading with Him to either take the bulimia or to take me—I couldn't stand to live another day as its victim.

Eventually, I began attending ministry school where I was certain I would find my freedom. It seemed to be the place where people were set free of addictions, and given a new chance at life. I was confident that this would be where I would find my answer. I was a worship leader, spending my days learning about God, studying the Bible, and even seeing miracles take place. On the outside everything seemed to line up with what a successful and happy Christian life should look like, but I still found myself in a seemingly never-ending battle with bulimia. Some days I would be able to resist it all day, only to come home and stay up until late into the night, once again stuffing myself with anything and everything I could find to eat. Other days I would wake up and go straight to the kitchen and begin bingeing and purging. One night I woke up at 2:00 a.m. and walked right to the kitchen to binge and purge half-awake—even in my deep sleep my heart hurt.

At that point in my life, I felt the weakest I ever had. I had never been suicidal, but I began fantasizing about not having to live anymore, about being free from bulimia, free from food, and free from myself. I couldn't understand why God hadn't set me free yet; why I would hear stories of other girls being radically delivered while I was still trapped and suffering. I had moved back in with my parents for the time, and my relationship with them became strained as they struggled with their feelings of helplessness. They had watched me destroy myself for so long, and their efforts felt useless. I had come to the point of accepting that this condition would eventually kill me and, truth be told, I hoped for it. I had fought for so long that my will and my hope had become depleted.

In the summer of 2012, something finally shifted. There were no fireworks, no great event or experience, but one day I lay in my bed with my throat throbbing from a long day of bingeing and purging, and something inside of me whispered, "This has to stop." I had thought that many times before, but this time a holy anger rose up inside of me. It was then that I realized that I was being violated. This wasn't a battle against myself, but a battle against the enemy, and I had allowed him to abuse me for too long. I jumped out of bed, grabbed my Bible, and began walking around my room declaring scriptures. "For it is written: I, Rihanna, am *more* than a conqueror!" "You've tried to hurt me, Satan, but God will use your evil for good, to save the lives of many people!" This went on for a few hours as I kept declaring truths over myself and my body. Looking back, I am sure I must have looked like a mad woman to anybody observing me, but I couldn't have cared less. Something inside me awakened as I began to see the ways bulimia had lied and stolen from me my entire life, and I was filled with a determination to win this battle.

The next day, I woke up still in fighter mode. I felt that the Lord had told me that I needed to fight both in the spiritual and the natural. I knew that the spiritual part of it would include the constant renewing of my mind by meditating on His words and Scriptures, as well as making declarations over myself. This was the easy part for me. The hard part was taking steps in the natural. I had to put myself on a meal plan with 2,000 calories per day. For some women 2,000 calories per day may sound high, but in my case this was necessary since my body had only ever known the cycle of starvation and bingeing, and I needed the calories to help my brain function and begin trusting that I wouldn't starve it again. What I found interesting is that when I was giving myself more calories, the desire to binge lessened dramatically.

I also had to discover my "why." Why did I want to recover? I got out a notecard and on one side wrote down what my life would look like in five years if I recovered. On the other side, I wrote down what my life would look like in five years if I didn't. As you can imagine, the difference was astounding. I kept that notecard with me, and used it many times to help me resist the urge to binge and purge because I now had a reason to keep getting healthier, and a clear picture of what would happen to my life if I were to give in.

As with any process, this journey wasn't over in one day. I didn't simply go to bed bulimic and wake up healed the next day. It was a step-by-step, day-by-day process. At first I was still bingeing and purging every day, even while implementing my new tools. However, instead of doing it six or eight times a day, it would only happen three to four times. Soon, it became two or three times, then one or two times, and then just once a day. I knew that shaming myself for every time I slipped up wouldn't bring me any healing, so instead I celebrated the moments that I resisted. There were many nights in which I would be praying and declaring Scriptures, only to find myself bingeing and purging within a few minutes. After years of abusing myself, I knew that feeling shame and guilt would only bring more harm, so I would immediately repent and go back into prayer.

As my journey of recovery went on, I had to stay sensitive and in tune with what God was telling me. I fully relied on Him to walk me through this recovery journey because I had never done this before and I knew that He knew the way. A few months into the process I had already come miles from where I started, but I was still struggling with unhealthy food obsessions, as well as some bingeing and purging. I knew that just being "mostly free" wasn't free enough. I pressed into God asking what my next step was. A few days later, someone told me about a study they had read in which they took students who weren't good at math and had them record themselves making positive statements like, "I am good at math," or, "Math is easy for me." They then had the students listen to their own recordings as they slept, and within a few weeks, their math skills dramatically improved. As she spoke, I knew that this was the answer from God that I was looking for. I went home and asked God to give me specific declarations that He wanted me to speak over myself. I then recorded them and for the next few months I listened to them every night in my sleep. It was supernatural how easy this next part of my journey became: I was filling my mind with truth while my insecurities didn't even get the chance to wake up and try to silence them.

November 10, 2012 was the last time that I made myself throw up. It still feels surreal to say that because my entire identity was wrapped up in bulimia for such a long time that I couldn't imagine a life without it. Even as I write this, I am brought to tears over the beauty of the redemption that God has given me. Along the way I lost count of how many times I begged and pleaded with God to deliver me. I would cry out and say, "If you heal me, I will never ask for or expect anything from you again." Looking back, I am so grateful that I was not delivered in a single moment. It was the journey out of bulimia that taught me just how strong I am. God is so gracious in not answering all of our prayers right away, and He continues to surpass my wildest expectations and heart's desires moment by moment in the process.

I am still on a journey into healthier living. It has been a process of having to relearn how to live now that bulimia has lost its power over me. In this process I find that I am learning something new about God, His incredible grace that restores us, life, and myself—every day. Grace has been explained as the empowering presence of God, and it is a key factor that Beni stresses over and over in teaching others how to journey into health. Grace has also been the key factor in my journey to freedom from eating disorders into health.

If you or someone you know is struggling with an eating disorder, there are many great resources available. Don't be afraid to reach out for help.

Visit http://www.nationaleatingdisorders.org for more information.

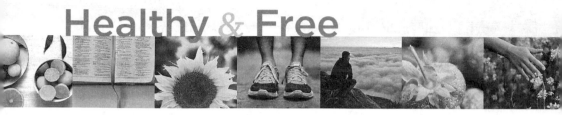

Healthy & Free

Chapter 8

Spirit Health

*Who ever knows what you're thinking and
planning except you yourself? The same with
God—except that he not only knows what
he's thinking, but he lets us in on it.*
—1 CORINTHIANS 2:11, MSG

In a previous chapter, I talked about the soul as the part of our being that looks toward earth. The spirit, on the other hand, is set on heavenly things and in the spirit life, one's gaze is turned toward Heaven. Since all health, life, and blessing come from Heaven and from our communion with God, it is of the highest importance that our spirit life is as strong as possible. I remember being told as a little girl that every person has a hole in their inner being that only Jesus can fill. I still believe that. How many of us have longed for something to fulfill us, and in that very search found Jesus? Once we found Him, our spirits became peaceful, and the search to fill the empty place inside was over. In my experience, a healthy spirit will impact the health of your physical body. This is another very important reason to understand how we can grow in taking care of our spirit.

Because I was born into a Christian family, Jesus has always been a part of my life. I was so young when I began to fall in love with Him that I don't even remember getting "saved." My life was lived *with* Him! I didn't know any other way. Having inherited a vibrant spiritual life from my parents, I can tell you that it is a wonderful and precious gift which I am deeply grateful for and treasure, but I also had to learn how to actively cultivate a healthy spirit life in an ongoing way, beyond my inheritance. My spirit life was radically changed in 1996 while visiting a church in Canada where I had an encounter with God that caused me to come alive in a way that I never had before. You know the story in the Bible when Jesus healed the blind man and at first he thought that the people he began to see were trees? Jesus then touched his eyes a second time and he was completely healed and could see accurately.[1] It wasn't that he couldn't see at all after the first time Jesus prayed, he just couldn't see clearly. When I encountered Jesus in that church in 1996 that was exactly how I felt, I began to see Jesus more clearly. When He touched me in that encounter, my spirit-man came into greater, abundant life. I am not saying that my spirit was dead before, but it just wasn't at its full capacity. God unlocked something within me and gave me a clear vision of Himself. Everything took on new life after this experience. I remember opening up my Bible, and experiencing Jesus through the words in a way that I had never felt before.

My spirit life changed dramatically as a result of this wonderful encounter. When I came home from that trip I began to do something that I had never really practiced before. I call it soaking. It is the art of focusing your gaze and attention on Him and adoring Him. I would take periods of time throughout my day and focus on paying attention to what He was saying and doing. Most of the time, I wouldn't say anything, sing, or even read the Bible. I would just play some worship music, lie on the floor, and commune with God. I would feel my spirit connect with His Holy Spirit, and I realized again just how incredibly rejuvenating it is to fellowship with God. I discovered that by doing this I was creating a strong, spiritual well in my inner being that would give me great internal strength and new health, which I also began to feel in my physical body.

Jesus is the Living Vine

I believe that keeping our spirit healthy is the most important part of our journey toward health and wellness. A healthy spirit is the foundation that everything else in our lives is built upon, and the source of all real strength. Building on this thought, when we put our spirit and the health of our spiritual life as a top priority, it can operate as a form of immune system. Hurts and hurdles will come our way, but the spiritual strength in God that comes through encountering and communing with Him is the main way that we overcome challenges. Conversely, if this part of our lives is weak then we won't thrive, and the hurts, hurdles, and challenges will be too much for us to conquer.

I know this from personal experience. I once had a student ask me how I handle being a leader in the face of the barrage of adversity and attacks that come to sabotage me. I told her my secret is I deal with these and other stressors by always trying to make sure that I spend time with God before I even leave the house in the morning. God is my rock, so whenever something tries to come against me, I know that I have Him, the solid anchor, holding me steady. Yes, it's true that from time to time I may sway a bit, but my peace comes from knowing that God will always be there to anchor me, protect me, and hold me. Jesus said,

> So step into life-union with me, for I have stepped into life-union with you. For as a branch severed from the vine will not bear fruit, so your life will be fruitless unless you live your life intimately joined to mine. I am the sprouting Vine and you're my branches. As you live in union with me as your source, fruitfulness will stream from within you, but

when you live separated from me you are powerless (John 15:4-5, TPT).

A Light Unto Our Path

Another important way to keep your spirit healthy is through thoroughly equipping yourself with the Bible. I have found that reading and quoting the Word of God out loud is a powerful tool against attacks, as well as a way to remind my inner being of God's truth. This is a personal tool, but it was further illustrated to me in a corporate setting in our church some time ago.

We had met a wonderful couple many years back, named Wesley and Stacey Campbell, who would read and declare the Scriptures out loud in their everyday lives. I was impacted by it. I will never forget the first time we had them come to Bethel, our church in Redding, California. Wesley got up to share and when he was done, he felt that the Lord was telling us all to get up out of our chairs, take our Bibles, and begin walking and reading the Scriptures out loud. Then, he told us to continue but to go outside. The whole crowd got up, took their Bibles, marched around the room, and excitedly exited out the back door into the parking lot. It became a powerful time as we began to proclaim the Word of God over our church and our city. I could feel the spiritual shift that it was causing both in our community as well as our church. It was a victorious moment, and a day that I'll always remember for the breakthrough that it brought to all of us.

Rihanna, the woman who recovered from bulimia, once shared with me that she had also heard Wesley and Stacey Campbell's message about praying and declaring the Scriptures over our lives and she too was deeply impacted by it. When she began her recovery journey, this practice became one of her most powerful tools. She would find Scriptures on victory and identity, and declare them over herself on a daily basis. She attributes a lot of her recovery to this message and the discipline of declaring God's Word out loud every day.

This is particularly important because it is in line with the very nature of the Bible; the Scriptures are the *rhema* Word of God. The word *rhema* implies a word that is spoken, an utterance: "A *rhema* is a verse or portion of Scripture that the Holy Spirit brings to our attention with application to a current situation or need for direction."[2] The Word of God is powerful and it is alive. These are some of my favorite verses that point to the power of the Scriptures, the way that they strengthen us spiritually, and, as a result, physically.

> *For the word of God is alive and powerful. It is sharper than the sharpest two-edged sword, cutting between soul and spirit, between joint and marrow. It exposes our innermost thoughts and desires* (Heb. 4:12, NLT).

> *My son, attend to my words; consent and submit to my sayings. Let them not depart from your sight; keep them in the center of your heart. For they are life to those who find them, healing and health to all their flesh* (Prov. 4:20-22).

> *You shall serve the Lord your God; He shall bless your bread and water, and will take sickness from your midst* (Exod. 23:25).

> *Be not wise in your own eyes; reverently fear and worship the Lord and turn [entirely] away from evil. It shall be health to your nerves and sinews, and marrow and moistening to your bones* (Prov. 3:7-8).

> *Heal me, O Lord, and I shall be healed; save me, and I shall be saved, for you are my praise* (Jer. 17:14, ESV).

> *Just then a woman who had suffered for twelve years with constant bleeding came up behind Him. She touched the fringe of His robe, for she thought, "If I can just touch His robe, I will be healed." Jesus turned around, and when he saw her he said, "Daughter, be encouraged! Your faith*

has made you well." And the woman was healed at that moment (Matt. 9:20-22, NLT).

As you can see, His words are powerful and they are sharper than any sword. What an amazing tool God has given to us to use. We can actually take the written Word of God, say it out loud, and He will cause it to actively work into our entire being! I personally feel that there is something about reading Scriptures out loud that releases their power. I believe that when you speak out loud the things of the Lord, you are letting the spirit realm, both the angels and demons, know where you stand, and as a result the atmosphere around you changes.

Not too long ago, a woman messaged me after seeing some of my posts regarding health and wellness. She was reaching out for help, and something inside me knew that I needed to keep in communication with her. Over the past few months she shared her story with me, and I was so moved by her willingness and dedication to renew her mind by using the power of declarations over her life. I asked her to share a bit of her story in the hopes that it may help you too.

> Seven pounds, two ounces. That's the least I have ever weighed. Although I struggled with a few extra pounds throughout my childhood, it never crossed my mind that I would eventually add over 450 pounds to my starting weight. Gain some, lose some. Gain it back, plus a few extra. This became the ruthless cycle of my life. I weighed 125 pounds when I got married and over 300 pounds just three years later when the marriage ended. Later in life, after a substantial weight gain, I worked for over a year to take off more than 250 pounds. After such an amazing feat it never crossed my mind that I would, indeed, put it all back on, plus a bit more.
>
> The perpetual hamster-wheel cycle of mustering up motivation, energetically engaging in the latest diet plan, losing a few pounds, losing focus, losing hope and ulti-mately giving up, eventually brought me to the unbelievable

point of weighing in at over 450 pounds. I am only 5' 2" with a small frame. How could this be? Why? What was I doing wrong? How could this keep happening? I am reasonably intelligent, and hold a couple of college degrees. I am active, and I am knowledgeable about health and diet. I love healthy food, and know what a healthy lifestyle looks like, spiritually, mentally, emotionally, and physically. I have a joyful, patient, and peaceful core character. I even swim for an hour most mornings at 4:30 A.M.

The self-discipline and willpower that it takes to lose as many pounds as I have, over the years of my life, is staggering. And yet, I, inadvertently and incessantly, return to a profusion of unhealthy choices, and each time they took me deeper down and further away from the Father's created intention for me.

And then, one day, something changed. Early in 2014, I began noticing Beni Johnson's posts on Facebook concerning overall health. Eventually, I mustered up the courage to send her a message and ask for some advice concerning my quandary. I was not only moved by her gracious reply, I now realize how this first encounter was a catalyst for a life-altering transformation. In addition to a concise list of very doable "Daily Dos" and "Definitely Don'ts," she referred me to a secular book called *The Gabriel Method* by Jon Gabriel, whose basic principle was more of a mind-body approach rather than just a simple, focus on food intake and exercise like most diet books. Although it was a secular book, it was clear that the concepts were identical to biblical principles—specifically the power of the spoken word.

Something clicked! I was reminded of the verse, "...be transformed by the renewing of your mind" (Rom. 12:2, NIV). The New Living version puts it like this: "...let

God transform you into a new person by changing the way you think."

I began to research, document, and journal Scriptures related to healing and health. Subsequently, I began to say them out loud, and literally proclaim them over myself on a regular basis. Coupled with better food choices and exercise, I began commanding my body and mind to line up with, and surrender to, the Kingdom principles on which I was created.

Before too long, I started noticing small but consistent changes. I no longer craved food-just-to-eat, especially in the evenings. I no longer had to fight off an insatiable appetite in stressful or highly emotional situations. It took a while for me to realize it, but, the most noticeable difference was that I was no longer obsessed with the usual stress and program progress of the self-will-driven weight-loss method. Something had changed.

The key—I had been overlooking the fact that based on God's Word I am a three-part being. Despite all my previous effort to obtain, and maintain, a healthy weight, this was the first time my mind, body, and spirit were coming into agreement. Balance.

Health-wise, from where I am, to where I need to end up, I still have a very long journey ahead. The good news is, my paradigm has shifted. Although the hamster-wheel syndrome was a dominant factor in my past, it has no part in my present or my future.

The vital, tangible power of the Truth so abundantly accessible in the letters left to us by our loving Father declare that I am no longer a slave to the lies that bring death and destruction.

I changed my mind!

Dewella

You see, diets did not work for her because she needed to get her soul, body, and spirit to come into alignment first. Lasting change has to begin within your heart.

So I have put together a list of Scriptures for you to begin reading out loud over your soul, body, and spirit. Join in faith with the promises of God and you'll experience another truth found in the Scriptures, that faith comes from hearing the Word of the Lord. In other words, God guarantees that you will be strengthened in your faith by declaring the Scriptures.

Physical Healing

O Lord my God, I cried to you for help, and you have healed me (Ps. 30:2, ESV).

Surely He has borne our griefs (sicknesses, weaknesses, and distresses) and carried our sorrows and pains [of punishment], yet we [ignorantly] considered Him stricken, smitten, and afflicted by God [as if with leprosy]. But He was wounded for our transgressions, He was bruised for our guilt and iniquities; the chastisement [needful to obtain] peace and well-being for us was upon Him, and with the stripes [that wounded] Him we are healed and made whole (Isa. 53:4-5).

He sends forth His word and heals them and rescues them from the pit and destruction (Ps. 107:20).

Then shall your light break forth like the morning, and your healing (your restoration and the power of a new life) shall spring forth speedily; your righteousness (your rightness, your justice, and your right relationship with God) shall go before you [conducting you to peace and prosperity], and the glory of the Lord shall be your rear guard (Isa. 58:8).

The eyes of the Lord are toward the [uncompromisingly] righteous and His ears are open to their cry. When the righteous cry for help, the Lord hears, and delivers them out of all their distress and troubles (Ps. 34:15,17).

God is our Refuge and Strength [mighty and impenetrable to temptation], a very present and well-proved help in trouble (Ps. 46:1).

The thief comes only in order to steal and kill and destroy. I came that they may have and enjoy life, and have it in abundance (to the full, till it overflows) (John 10:10).

Spirit Healing

Therefore, [there is] now no condemnation (no adjudging guilty of wrong) for those who are in Christ Jesus, who live [and] walk not after the dictates of the flesh, but after the dictates of the Spirit. For the law of the Spirit of life [which is] in Christ Jesus [the law of our new being] has freed me from the law of sin and of death (Rom. 8:1-2).

But if Christ lives in you, [then although] your [natural] body is dead by reason of sin and guilt, the spirit is alive because of [the] righteousness [that He imputes to you] (Rom. 8:10).

One thing have I asked of the Lord, that will I seek, inquire for, and [insistently] require: that I may dwell in the house of the Lord [in His presence] all the days of my life, to behold and gaze upon the beauty [the sweet attractiveness and the delightful loveliness] of the Lord and to meditate, consider, and inquire in His temple (Ps. 27:4).

You will show me the path of life; in your presence is fullness of joy, at your right hand there are pleasures forevermore (Ps. 16:11, NKJV).

Emotional Healing

He heals the brokenhearted and binds up their wounds [curing their pains and their sorrows] (Ps. 147:3).

Do not fret or have any anxiety about anything, but in every circumstance and in everything, by prayer and petition (definite requests), with thanksgiving, continue to make your wants known to God. And God's peace [shall be yours, that tranquil state of a soul assured of its salvation through Christ, and so fearing nothing from God and being content with its earthly lot of whatever sort that is, that peace] which transcends all understanding shall garrison and mount guard over your hearts and minds in Christ Jesus (Phil. 4:6-7).

Why are you cast down, O my inner self? And why should you moan over me and be disquieted within me? Hope in God and wait expectantly for Him, for I shall yet praise Him, my Help and my God (Ps. 42:5).

You have turned my mourning into dancing for me; you have put off my sackcloth and girded me with gladness (Ps. 30:11).

The Lord is close to those who are of a broken heart and saves such as are crushed with sorrow for sin and are humbly and thoroughly penitent (Ps. 34:18).

This is my comfort and consolation in my affliction: that your word has revived me and given me life (Ps. 119:50).

Be strong, courageous, and firm; fear not nor be in terror before them, for it is the Lord your God Who goes with you; He will not fail you or forsake you (Deut. 31:6).

For God did not give us a spirit of timidity (of cowardice, of craven and cringing and fawning fear), but [He has given us a spirit] of power and of love and of calm and well-balanced mind and discipline and self-control (2 Tim. 1:7).

And be constantly renewed in the spirit of your mind [having a fresh mental and spiritual attitude], and put on the new nature (the regenerate self) created in God's image, [Godlike] in true righteousness and holiness (Eph. 4:23-24).

You will guard him and keep him in perfect and constant peace whose mind [both its inclination and its character] is stayed on you because he commits himself to you, leans on you, and hopes confidently in you (Isa. 26:3).

If you commit to taking three verses a day and declaring them over your physical, emotional, and spiritual health, I am confident that that you will see an amazing change in your life. Faith and hope will begin to rise up within your very being. As you read them, allow yourself to connect with the meaning and substance of the words because there is power and healing within them that will change your life.

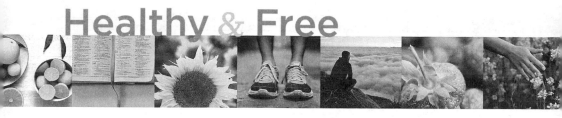

Epilogue

"God created it. Jesus died for it. The Holy
Spirit lives in it. I'd better take care of it."
—RICK WARREN

As you can see, the journey of health and wellness is just that—a journey. It is filled with explorations, wandering, victories, and moments
when you have to retrace your steps to get back on track.

And as you can see from my story, it hasn't always been easy.
There were moments when I had to sit back and remind myself of my
"why." I had to align my thoughts with Heaven's, allow myself to see
His perspective, and then declare His truth.

My prayer is that in the moments when you feel like giving up, you
will instead lean on the strength of God to pull you through. Remember, He is more dedicated to seeing you succeed than you are. Health
was His idea from the beginning. He made your body, soul, and
spirit—those three parts of your being that are all connected—and

when they are healthy and in harmony with each other, you will experience wellness. Remember, God designed us as His beautiful piece of art. He made us to function in a way that brings Him glory.

Don't be afraid to start small. Take those baby steps, and you will find that they will turn into victories. Those victories will lead to even bigger ones. I have faith for you—overcomer—you were born to be healthy and free!

To your health,
Beni Johnson

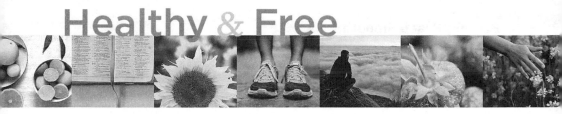

Healthy & Free

Recipes

Healthy foods do not have to be flavorless and bland. One of my passions is cooking and baking with healthy foods because I love being able to enjoy the outcome knowing that it is healthy for my body. Here are a few recipes to help get you started.

Smoothies

Green Lemonade Smoothie

2 handfuls chopped romaine

1 tablespoon raw organic honey

1 peeled lemon

½ green apple

½ avocado

Combine all ingredients in a blender with ½ cup filtered water or coconut water. Blend.

Protein Peach Smoothie

1 small peach

¼ cup raspberries

¼ cup protein powder

¼ cup raw chai protein powder

1 cup flaxseed milk

½ cup filtered water

½ teaspoon maca powder

1 teaspoon magnesium

2 packs Stevia

Combine all ingredients in a blender. Blend and enjoy.

Maca Energy Drink

12–16 ounces coconut water (use another juice if you can't use coconut)

⅓ teaspoon of maca

1½ teaspoon of Spirulina

1 tablespoon of raw cocoa powder (I use fat-free Wondercocoa, 99.7% caffeine-free)

small handful of goji berries or ½ to 1 teaspoon of goji berry powder

Blend and drink. (I put a few drops of Stevia in mine.)[1]

Breakfast

Homemade Granola

6 cups soaked nuts (I prefer almonds and cashews)

½ cup raw honey

2 tablespoons maca powder (optional)

¾ cup dates

¼ cup flax seeds

1 tablespoon vanilla

¼ cup buckwheat flour (optional)

½ cup hemp seeds

¼ cup chia seeds

Soak the nuts in filtered water for at least four hours, or overnight. Drain the water and put the nuts in a food processor with the honey, maca, dates, flax seed, and vanilla. Combine them by pulsing the blender, but be careful not to process too much; you want it to retain its texture. Put that nut mixture into a big bowl and mix in the hemp and chia seeds. Spread the mixture out onto dehydrator trays and dehydrate at least 12e hours at 118 degrees.

Acai Bowl

1 packet of acai powder (or 1 tablespoon)

2 tablespoons chia seeds

1 cup water or organic apple juice

Blend ingredients together and refrigerate for one or two hours. Once it's of a pudding consistency, add your favorite fruit with some healthy granola.

Quinoa Protein Pancakes

2 eggs

2 cups almond milk

1½ teaspoons lemon juice

4 tablespoons coconut oil

2 cups almond flour

½ cup hazelnut flour

2 tablespoon palm sugar

2 teaspoons baking powder

1 teaspoon baking soda

1 teaspoon salt

2 cups cooked red quinoa

1 tablespoon tapioca flour

Place the milk in a small bowl and pour in the lemon juice. Stir once and allow to sit for five minutes. Combine flour, sugar, baking powder, baking soda, and salt in a bowl and mix together. Place the eggs in a mixing bowl and beat with a wire whisk. Add the coconut oil, dry ingredients, and milk to the eggs and mix until combined. Add the quinoa to the batter and mix until combined—do not over-mix. Heat a griddle to medium or medium-high and grease with coconut oil. Pour the batter onto the hot griddle (about ¼ cup per pancake) and allow to cook for a minute or so, or until the top of the pancake has bubbled up and the sides are cooked. Flip the pancake over and finish cooking on the other side for another 30 seconds.

Lunch

Tuna Salad Lettuce Wraps

These are a great go-to for lunch on the go that won't sabotage your health! Also try with shredded chicken for something different.

1 can albacore tuna

handful red grapes

1 stalk celery

Himalayan salt

pepper

cumin

1½ tablespoons Veganaise

Combine tuna and Veganaise. Slice red grapes and celery into small pieces and add to tuna mix. Season with Himalayan salt, pepper, and cumin to taste. Top onto whole romaine lettuce leaves and enjoy!

Chicken Strips

This is a great healthy alternative for chicken nuggets. Little ones are fans as well as grownups!

3 boneless chicken breasts

2 eggs

1 cup almond flour

1 teaspoon garlic powder

1 teaspoon paprika

salt and pepper to taste

Preheat oven to 425 degrees. Cut chicken in long, inch-wide slices. Combine almond flour, garlic powder, paprika, and salt, and pepper. Whip eggs. Place one chicken strip in the eggs, then coat in dry mixture. Place on parchment paper in oven and cook for 10 minutes or until chicken is thoroughly cooked.

Protein Peppers

½ pound ground chicken (or ground meat of your choice)

1 onion, chopped

1 celery stalk, chopped

1 can tomato paste

1 bag mini peppers

salt and pepper to taste

Sauté chicken with salt and pepper until fully cooked. Drain any extra fat. Add chopped onion and celery with tomato paste and mix. Slice the tops off of the peppers and take out any seeds. Stuff peppers with chicken mixture. Place in oven under a low broiler until the peppers are soft.

Dinner

Gluten and Grain-Free Pizza

For the crust:

> 2 eggs
>
> 1½ cups almond flour
>
> 3 tablespoons liquid ghee (or organic, "grassfed" butter)
>
> ½ teaspoon gluten-free baking powder
>
> 1 teaspoon salt
>
> ½ teaspoon ground basil
>
> ½ teaspoon powdered garlic

For the topping:

¼ cup tomato paste

1 teaspoon salt

½ teaspoon ground basil

meat of your choice

handful of diced tomatoes

handful of mixed olives (black and green)

about ½ cup cheese of your choice

Combine and mix ingredients for the crust and set in the fridge for at least 30 minutes. Once chilled, place between two pieces of parchment paper and use a pizza roller to roll out the dough. Bake dough for five minutes at 350 degrees. Remove from the oven and spread with tomato paste, sprinkle with salt, basil, and place all the other ingredients on top. Bake for an additional ten or fifteen minutes at the same temperature.

Raw Pad Thai

Vegetables:

 6 cups shredded cabbage

 4 large carrots

 1 bunch cilantro, finely chopped

 2 large zucchini, thinly sliced

 1 large yellow pepper

Sauce:

 1 cup raw almond butter

 4 tablespoons fresh ginger

 1 cup water

 8 tablespoons fresh lemon juice

 ½ cup pure maple syrup

 6 tablespoons Nama Shoyu sauce

 8 teaspoons sesame oil

 1 hot pepper (optional)

 2–3 cloves of garlic

Base:

meat of 2–3 young coconuts

Topping:

handful of cashews

sprouted greens

Prepare vegetables and mix in a bowl. Combine the sauce ingredients and put in a blender and blend until of creamy consistency. On a plate, place the coconut meat and top with the fresh vegetables. Then pour sauce over the vegetables and mix until coated. Top with chopped cashews and your choice of sprouted greens.

Zoodles

"Zoodles" (otherwise known as zucchini noodles) are my favorite go-to when I need something quick, easy, and healthy! You can do so much with zoodles; they are guaranteed to never get boring! I recommend investing in a spiral vegetable slicer (also known as a "spirulizer"), which you can find online. Here is my favorite simple recipe.

> 2 large zucchinis, spirulized
>
> ¼ cup organic olive oil
>
> 1 cup chopped grape tomatoes
>
> ½ lemon
>
> salt and pepper to taste

Spirulize the zucchini and place in bowl. Add grape tomatoes and olive oil and mix. Squeeze ½ lemon over the top and add salt and pepper to taste.

Desserts

Protein *"Ice Cream"*

> 3 cups almond milk
>
> 3 scoops organic protein powder
>
> 2 tablespoons cocoa
>
> Stevia to taste

Combine ingredients and put into an ice cream maker until it reaches ice cream consistency. Top with freshly chopped fruit, dates or nuts.

Gluten-Free Ginger Oatmeal Cookies

> 2 ripe bananas
>
> 2 tablespoons maple syrup
>
> 2 tablespoons grapeseed or coconut oil

1½ cups gluten-free rolled oats

2 tablespoons ground flax seeds

1½ teaspoons cinnamon

2 dates, chopped

1 tablespoon fresh ginger, chopped

¼ cup goji berries

¼ cup cranberries

¼ cup fair-trade dark chocolate

Preheat oven to 350 degrees. Mash bananas until fully smooth. Add maple syrup and grapeseed oil, and stir. In a separate bowl, combine oats, flax seeds, cinnamon, dates, ginger, goji berries, and cranberries. Stir in banana mix and whisk until fully blended. Add chopped dark chocolate. Place onto cookie sheet lined with parchment paper or greased, and bake in oven for 10 minutes.

Raw Chocolate Pudding

2 cups of fresh coconut meat (or I use coconut strings I find in my local Asian store)

2 cups coconut strings

¾ cup coconut water

½ cup maple syrup

¾ cup raw agave nectar

½ cup cocoa powder

2 tablespoons vanilla

¼ teaspoon sea salt

Combine all ingredients in blender and blend until it reaches a smooth, pudding consistency. Refrigerate and let it sit for 2–3 hours before eating.

Miscellaneous

The Master Tonic

This keeps your immune system healthy, especially in the winter. It is packed full of natural antibiotics and anti-inflammatories.

1 part fresh chopped garlic

1 part fresh chopped onion

1 part fresh grated ginger root

1 part fresh grated horseradish root

1 part fresh chopped cayenne peppers or any hot peppers seasonally available

Raw, unfiltered apple cider vinegar

(I recommend using only fresh and preferably organically grown herbs if possible, as this will make the most potent and effective Master Tonic. Substitute dried herbs only in an emergency if fresh is unavailable.)

Fill a glass Mason jar three-quarters full of the above fresh chopped and grated herbs. (Wear gloves when chopping the hot peppers.) Fill the jar to the top with raw apple cider vinegar. Close the lid tightly and shake, leave on countertop, shake at least once a day for two weeks, and then filter the Master Tonic mixture through a clean piece of cloth, bottle and label. Store in the refrigerator. You can shake this tonic every time you walk by it, a minimum of once per day.

Hibiscus Kombucha

Kombucha is loaded with enzymes and probiotics, which help keep our digestive systems happy and healthy. I can't sing its praises enough! This is my favorite recipe that I often make at home.

4 green teabags, decaffeinated

¼ cup dried hibiscus

1 cup organic sugar

3 quarts filtered water

½ cup of kombucha

1 organic scoby (starter culture)

Bring the water to a boil, then turn off the heat and add the sugar. Stir until the sugar is fully dissolved. Add the teabags and hibiscus. Let it sit for 30 minutes, then remove the teabags and let it cool thoroughly. Once cooled, pour into a gallon jar and add the half cup of kombucha and the scoby. Put a paper towel or thin towel over the top. Do not put the lid on. Put the jar in a dark place for seven to nine days and do not move it. After, remove the scoby. (You should now have a baby scoby, too, which you can use for your next batch. The old scoby is still good and can be used over again as well.)

Pour this juice into jars with lids to prepare for the second ferment, during which time juices or ginger can be added to the recipe. (I use ginger juice and at times add fruit juices as well.) A little goes a long way; add only about two or three *tablespoons* of juice. Place the lids on the containers and keep them on the counter for three days, then refrigerate and enjoy!

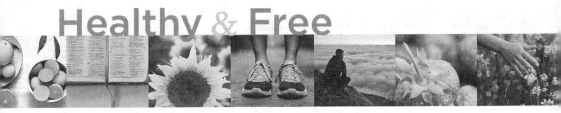

Questions and Answers

Q: What's a good essential oil for inflammation or muscle pain?

A: I use peppermint oil by Young Living. I use it all the time and not only does it help with inflammation, it also helps with allergies. I put a couple drops in my hand, rub my hands together, and place my palm on the back of my neck. Then I inhale it three times. For muscle relief, put a couple of drops in your palm, rub your hands together, and rub into the place of soreness. You can also put a couple of drops into a good lotion or coconut oil and rub on those sore muscles.

There are more oils, of course, and you can Google them, but peppermint is the one that works best for me. (They always know when I'm at the gym because I use it right in the locker room.) Another product that I just got from Young Living is called Ortho Sport massage oil. It is working really well too.

Q: I bought some cinnamon essential oil. What is its benefit?

A: Cinnamon bark is an anti-inflammatory, a powerful antibacterial, and a stomach protectant (against ulcers). It's also an anti-parasitic (worms) and is used for cardiovascular disease, infectious diseases, digestive complaints, and warts. How to use: I dilute one part oil with four parts pure oil (such as olive oil or coconut) and place right at location of the problem or on the flex points on your feet. You may also take it as a supplement, putting a drop or two in a vegetable capsule. I wouldn't recommend you taking it on an empty stomach though, because it's what is called a "hot oil"; be careful when ingesting it.

Q: *Why is protein so good for you?*

A: It is a component of every cell in your body. In fact, hair and nails are mostly made of protein. Your body uses it to build and repair tissue and you need it to make enzymes, hormones, and other body chemicals. It is also an important building block of bones, muscles, cartilage, skin, and blood. Like carbohydrates and fat, protein is a "macronutrient," meaning that you need relatively large amounts of it to stay healthy. (Vitamins and minerals, which you need in small quantities only, are called "micronutrients.") Your body does not store protein as it does carbohydrates and fat, so it has no reservoir to draw from when you're running low. Consuming high-protein foods has many benefits, including:

- speeding recovery after exercise
- reducing muscle loss
- building lean muscle
- helping you maintain a healthy weight
- curbing hunger

Having protein in your diet, especially as you get older, will help in maintaining your muscles mass. (As you age, you lose muscle.)

Q: *How can you build muscle after the age of 45 if you have never worked out in your life?*

A: It's never too late! When you are around 40, you start to lose muscle and you lose more the older you get. That is why you see people who are older with prominent bellies. Muscle burns fat! So, how to gain muscle? All the sources I've consulted say the way to gain muscle is to lift weights. Many women are afraid to lift weights because they are afraid they will get too muscular and have "ugly man muscles," but I can tell you that is not going to happen unless you are taking drugs for that reason. You will have to work hard at the gym, though; work different muscles groups throughout the week and give those muscle groups at least 48 hours to rest between workouts. In other words, on back and bicep day, work those muscles hard, and then make sure you rest them for two days before you work them again. I go to the gym three days a week, working two sets of muscle groups each day: Monday—chest and biceps, Tuesday—triceps and back, Fridays—shoulders and legs. I also mix in some core work and abs-building.

Eating protein is also important. Right after a workout (normally within 15 minutes) is the best time to eat protein or drink protein shakes. It will help your muscles grow. If you can, I recommend getting a trainer for a week to help set you up on a routine.

Q: How do you lose weight when you have adrenal fatigue or PCOS (polycystic ovary syndrome)?

A: Boy, I know this one well. What's more important than losing weight is that you heal first. When I went through adrenal fatigue, I had to cut my exercise way down. I would go for easy walks and incorporate some stretching. After I got better, I was able to go to the gym again. But, you *must* allow yourself to heal first, because if you don't you will continue to crash and burn. You might feel good after a workout, but you will find yourself crashing; it's just a vicious cycle. Get well and give yourself some grace for this season of healing. It's the same with the PCOS—you need to heal first. Here are some natural ways to promote healing:

- Low-glycemic-index carbohydrates should be balanced with sufficient protein.

- Intake of saturated fats should be reduced.

- Dairy products should be avoided or limited.
- Additives, food chemicals and preservatives should be avoided.
- Alcohol and caffeine should be avoided.
- Sugar should be avoided.
- Two liters of filtered water should be consumed daily.
- Omega-3 essential fatty acids should be included in diet.

To incorporate these changes into your lifestyle, I would suggest going on a paleo diet.

Q: *What's the best remedy for sugar cravings?*

A: I juice greens such as romaine and kale. Those dark greens seem to cut the craving for me. I make a green lemonade juice with a juicer or blender (using the blender keeps the fiber in the drink). Here is the recipe:

5–6 leaves of romaine and kale (you may need to use more)

1 peeled lemon.

1 green apple (remove seeds)

filtered water for smoothness

Blend and drink in the mornings.

Where supplements are concerned, here are a couple of online articles that have good suggestions. (Although Stevia is suggested, you may need to stay away from that if you are in your child-bearing years.)

- "Herbal Remedies for Sugar Cravings" at Livestrong. com, http://www.livestrong.com/article/107164-herbal -remedies-sugar-cravings/.
- "5 Supplements that Reduce Sugar Cravings" at 3 Fat Chicks on a Diet, http://www.3fatchicks.com/5- supplements-that-reduce -sugar-cravings/.

Q: What are your thought on vaccines and fluoride?

A: I personally recommend neither. Concerning the vaccines, I tell people that it's your call and that you need to do what your heart is telling you to do. I've read too much information and heard too many frightening stories to ever take a vaccine. As far as fluoride is concerned, I stay as far away from it as possible, because it's a poison, a toxic chemical. I use a good water filter that takes out the fluoride in the tap water, and I use a non-fluoride brand of toothpaste that has xylitol in it, which helps fight cavities. Here are a couple of products:

- Natural Healing Tooth Powder from DHerbs.com, http://dherbs.com/store/natural-healing-tooth-powder -p-364.html#.VDV6_0R9lec.

- Daily Oral Therapy from Dr. Schulze's American Botanical Pharmacy, https://www.herbdoc.comh (this tooth and gum polish is what I use).

Q: How do you maintain a healthy diet on a tight budget?

A: By planning ahead. I had two boys and I used to say that one of them had two empty legs and he filled them up all day long. We ate a lot of tuna and pasta back then. You could serve brown rice with butter on it (add some hemp seeds to it for protein). You could go in with friends and buy a side of beef (preferably from a naturally grass-fed animal). Buying in bulk is always the best way. If you have a busy schedule, take one day a week and make homemade meals ahead of time, aiming for things you can save in the freezer or refrigerator. Shoestring budget healthy grocery list:

- Brown rice

- Steamed fresh vegetables

- Organic butter (a farmers market is a good place to buy)

- Hemp seeds (a good source of protein)

- Avocadoes (They are a complete food!)
- Almond butter (a good source of fat and protein)

Better yet, make your own almond or any nut butter. Here is a recipe site for nut butters: Tasty Yummies at http://tasty-yummies .com/2014/03/18/how-to-make-homemade-nut-butters/. (The site recommends that you soak and dehydrate the nuts first, but you don't have to.) If you don't have a food processor, ask around and see if you can borrow one from a friend.

Q: Why is kombucha good for me?

A: Homemade kombucha is a great way to get both probiotics and enzymes, and is very cheap to make. Probiotics provide "good flora" in your gut; good flora gets disrupted when you take antibiotics (catch the "anti" part) and for other more general reasons. Cooking foods kills all the natural enzymes, and we need enzymes to digest our foods. Kombucha is one of my favorite drinks. My body craves it. If you go to Pinterest (search Beni Johnson), you will find some good recipes. I especially like the hibiscus recipe.

Q: Is it OK for women to take whey protein?

A: If you can handle whey, then go for it. I would suggest that you look at this site and decide which type of protein might be best for you. Non-denatured whey is purer. I did at one time take a non-denatured brand (Standard Process, a great company). You can find more information at the PaleoHacks website: http://paleohacks.com/whey/ undenatured-whey-protein-vs-whey-protein-isolate-4187.

Q: How do I change my lifestyle (eating, exercise)? It seems as if I don't have the time.

A: Sit down and figure out your "why," your reason to make changes. You don't have to go to the gym or become a vegan. This is your journey and you have to figure out what's important to you and your family. Educate yourself. If you have to put yourself on a schedule, then do that. Look for DVDs and online exercise programs that you can do in your own home. Read books and find good websites. Some resources I suggest include: *The Seven Pillars of Health,* by Dr. Don Colbert, the "Juice Lady," Cherie Calbom's site (http://www.juiceladycherie.com), and author Jordon Rubin's books. I always suggest eating a paleo diet, and for guidance I recommend the series of cookbooks by Danielle Walker called *Against All Grain.*

Q: *What's wrong with dairy?*

A: Commercial milks, used for the typical type of dairy products that you find in your grocery store, contain growth hormones and/or antibiotics that are given to the cows. In addition, the grass they eat or the other foods that they get have pesticides in them, and it all goes into the milk. Personally, I don't want to be drinking or eating growth hormones, antibiotics, or pesticides. I recommend using raw, organic forms of these products. Here is a good source of understanding on this issue at Dr. Joseph Mercola's website: http://www.mercola.com/article/milk/no-milk.htm.

Q: *What quick, at-home workouts would you recommend for a busy person?*

A: I would Google "workout videos" on your computer. I've found good 30-minute workouts using the bands (which you can find on the store of my blog site, Grandmas With Muscles—grandmaswithmuscles.com). There's so much out there on the Internet that will help you get your exercise on. I have posted some at-home workouts on my blog that you can do with some basic equipment.

Q: *What are some healthy dairy-free recipes?*

A: I would recommend looking into some paleo recipes because they omit dairy while using healthy sugars and flours. Danielle Walker has written a series of books called *Against All Grain* that I use when I need some inspiration (website as well at againstallgrain.com). Again, you can search online to get some ideas. Whenever I want a good paleo recipe, I look online.

Q: What are your thoughts on CoQ$_{10}$?

A: I take it every day! I always make sure that I get a good and pure brand and not just something you can pick up at the corner drugstore. Health food stores usually carry good brands that are organic.

Q: What do you recommend for healthy pregnancy, childbirth, and postpartum?

A: I suggest everything that applies to having a healthy life, period. I highly recommend the book, *The Seven Pillars of Health,* by Dr. Don Colbert. Be sure to eat well during and after your pregnancy. It is important to help keep your body in balance. Exercise is one way of keeping the blues away after your pregnancy. Just make sure you talk with your doctor about when and how much you can do. Another tip I've learned from some of my gal friends that have been pregnant more recently than I have is to drink raw milk (from a reliable, organic source). Here is just one website, Healing Our Children, of many that encourages drinking raw milk during pregnancy: http://www.healingourchildren.net/Pregnancy_Diet/raw_milk_pregnancy.htm.

Q: What is a good alternative to beef?

A: Beef has some great health benefits such as iron and a good source of fat. However, if you are looking for a good protein alternative, I recommend http://www.thehealthyhomeeconomist.com/master-tonic-natural-flu-antiviral/. Fish, chicken, hemp seeds or hemp protein powder, chia seeds, cranberries and peas are good alternatives for your daily protein.

Q: How would you suggest dealing with menopause?

A: There are several natural and healthy supplements you can take. One is maca. (Use ½ teaspoon a day in or on your food. I think it tastes better in a shake or blended juice.) Another product that I can't live without is the liquid vitamin Sea Aloe. This is not just for menopause. I recommend this to young girls, moms, and anybody who feels out of control with their emotions. I have actually had husbands message me to thank me for helping their wives. (I order mine from Nature's Liquids at: http://www .myseaaloe.com/default.aspx?ovtid=287&spnid=92330016&gclid=CNC -strirMECFVFgMgodFGkAbQ. Make sure you order the red bottle.)

The thing I've found that works best is eating right. If you consume sugar or even a lot of fruit, look out for those hot flashes. I avoid eating any carbs or fruit right before bed because it increases the hot flashes at night. BBC Good Food has a great read on menopause and food (the only thing I don't recommend is the soy part): http://www.bbcgoodfood .com/howto/guide/eat-beat-menopause. Another recommendation that I would add to the above article is to add more fiber to your diet. It prevents constipation while lowering cholesterol and blood glucose, and it addresses many other health concerns that come with menopause. Using fiber-rich products to replace refined carbohydrates such as pasta and white bread can make your system run much smoother.

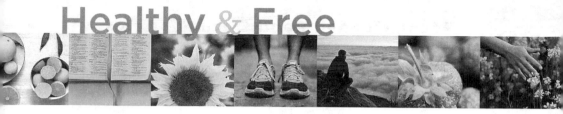

Healthy & Free

Resources

Recommended Product Brands

- Sea Aloe http://www.myseaaloe.com/default.aspx
- Pure Encapsulation http://www.pureencapsulations.com/
- Standard Process
- Garden of Life http://www.gardenoflife.com/
- Organic India Turmeric http://organicindiausa.com/organic-india-turmeric-formula/
- Fit Aid Fitness Drink www.drinkfitaid.com
- Fluoride Water Filter www.store.seychelle.com
- PH Strips (To test acidic/alkalized levels in body) https://www.microessentiallab.com/ProductInfo/F03-WIDRG-000130-JUD.aspx
- Organic Buffalo Meat www.wildideabuffalo.com/
- Young Living Oils www.youngliving.com/beni4health
- Vital Proteins http://www.vitalproteins.com/

Recommended Food Documentaries

- *Food Inc.*
- *Hungry for Change*
- *Fat, Sick, and Nearly Dead*
- *Forks over Knives*
- *Food Matters*
- *Super Size Me*

Recommended Reading

- *The Seven Pillars of Health* by Dr. Colbert, http://sevenpillarsofhealth.com/
- *The Makers Diet* by Jordin Rubin, http://www.makers-diet.net/
- *Thyroid Healthy* by Susan Cohen, http://suzycohen.com/
- *The Gabriel Method* by Jon Gabriel, http://www.thegabrielmethod.com/
- *Earthing: The Most Important Health Discovery Ever?* by Clinton Ober, Steven Sinatra, and Martin Zucker
- *Water: For Health, for Healing, for Life: You're Not Sick, You're Thirsty!* by F. Batmanghelidj
- *Switch Your Brain On* by Dr Caroline Leaf, http://drleaf.com/
- *Declarations* by Steve Backlund, http://ignitinghope.com/
- *Let's Just Laugh at That* by Steve Backlund, http://ignitinghope.com/
- *The Passion Translation,* www.thepassiontranslation.com
- *Natural to Supernatural Health* by David Herzog

- *Intuitive Eating* by Evelyn Tribole and Elyse Resch, https://www.intuitiveeating.com
- *The Hormone Reset Diet* by Sara Gottfried
- *The New ME Diet* by Jade Teta and Keoni Teta

Recommended Blogs

- *Grandmas With Muscles* www.grandmaswithmuscles.com
- *The Juice Lady* www.juiceladycherie.com/Juice
- *Against All Grains* www.againstallgrain.com
- *Brittany Angell* http://brittanyangell.com/every-last-crumb/
- *The Whole Food Diary* www.thewholefooddiary.com
- *Unprocess Your Foods* www.bydash.com
- *Food Babe* http://foodbabe.com/
- *Metabolic Effect* http://www.metaboliceffect.com/

To find a practicing naturopath or homeopathic doctor in your area visit the website of the American Association of Naturopathic Physicians: http://www.naturopathic.org/AF_MemberDirectory.asp?version=2.

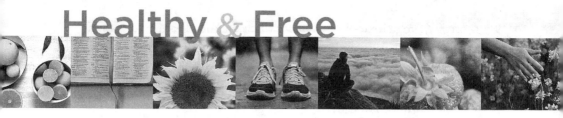

Notes

Chapter 1: The Journey

1. "What is Adrenal Fatigue?" Future Formulations, www.adrenalfatigue
   .org

Chapter 2: Soul Health

1. "Trichotomous v. Dichotomous views of Man," Christianity Stack
   Exchange, http://christianity.stackexchange.com/questions/8847/
   trichotomous -vs-dichotomous-views-of-man/8887#8887.
2. "Jessica's Daily Affirmation," Youtube, June 16, 2009, http://www
   .youtube.com/watch?v=qR3rK0kZFkg.
3. Caroline Leaf, "The Science of Love, Dr. Caroline Leaf, September
   29, 2011, http://drleaf.com/blog/the-science-of-love/.
4. Caroline Leaf, *Who Switched Off My Brain* (Nashville, Thomas
   Nelson, 2009), 19.
5. Jon Gabriel, *The Gabriel Method* (New York, Atria Books, 2008), 15.
6. Ibid., 33.
7. Caroline Leaf, "Toxic Thoughts," *Dr. Caroline Leaf*, http://drleaf.com/
   about/toxic-thoughts/.
8. Ibid.

9. "21 Days to a Toxic-Free Mind," Switch on Your Brain International, http://21daybraindetox.com.

10. John J. Parsons, "Thoughts on Repentence," Hebrew for Christians, http://www.hebrew4christians.com/Holidays/Fall_Holidays/Elul/ Teshuvah/teshuvah.html.

11. Jack Graham, "What Does it Mean to 'Repent'?" Jesus.org, http:// www.jesus.org/following-jesus/repentance-faith-and-salvation/what -does-it-mean-to-repent.html.

12. West's Encyclopedia of American Law, ed. 2005, Encyclopedia.com, s.v. "Declaration," http://www.encyclopedia.com/topic/Declaration .aspx.

13. Steve Blacklund, *Declarations, Unlocking Your Future* (Redding, Calif.: Igniting Hope Ministries, 2013), 1.

14. Pamela Gerloff, "You're Not Laughing Enough, and That's No Joke," *The Possibility Paradigm blog*, posted June 20, 2011, Psychology Today, http://www.psychologytoday.com/blog/the-possibility-paradigm/201106/youre-not-laughing -enough-and-thats-no-joke

15. Melinda Smith and Jeanne Segal, "Laughter is the Best Medicine," Helpguide.org, updated June 2015, http://www.helpguide.org/articles/ emotional-health/laughter-is-the-best-medicine.htm.

Chapter 3: God's Art

1. Genesis 1:26–28.

2. Luke 12:7.

4.1: Hydration

1. "The Water in You," U.S. Department of the Interior, updated May 5, 2015, http://water.usgs.gov/edu/propertyyou.html.

2. Don Colbert, *The Seven Pillars of Health* (Lake Mary, Fla.: Charisma House, 2007), 7.

3. Anne Marie Helmenstine, "How Much of Your Body is Water?" About. com, http://chemistry.about.com/od/waterchemistry/f/How-Much-Of -Your-Body-Is-Water.htm.

4. David Herzog, *Natural to Supernatural Health* (Sedona, Ariz.: DHE Publishing, 2010), 30.

5. "Functions of Water in Your Body," Magnation Corporation, http:// www.moreplant.com/health/functions-of-water.php.

6.   Ibid.

7.   On a side note, many believe that it is important to limit your water intake while eating a meal to only about eight ounces, as it might interfere with the digestion process by reducing your stomach acids. A good rule of thumb is to drink no less than 20 minutes before your meal, and then wait for another 20 minutes afterward before having more.

8.   F. Batmanghelidj, *You're Not Sick, You're Thirsty* (New York: Warner, 2003), 32.

9.   Colbert, *The Seven Pillars of Health*, 15.

10. For more information, I recommend reading the 1988 book, *Troubled Waters on Tap*, by Duff Conacher.

11. Colbert, *The Seven Pillars of Health*, 17.

12. Suzann Wang, "Toothpaste Woes: Fluoride's Dark Side," Green Health Spot, http://www.greenhealthspot.com/2008/01/toothpaste-woes.html.

4.2: The Power of Sleep

1.   Kendra Cherry, "The Four Stages of Sleep," About.com, http://psychology.about.com/od/statesofconsciousness/a/SleepStages.htm.

2.   Diana L. Walcutt, "Stages of Sleep," PsychCentral.com, January 30, 2013, http://psychcentral.com/lib/stages-of-sleep/0002073.

3.   Laura Schocker, "Your Body Does Incredible Things When You Aren't Awake," *Huffington Post,* March 7, 2014, http://www.huffingtonpost.com/2014/03/07/your-body-does-incredible_n_4914577.html.

4.   Ibid.

5.   "What Happens When You Sleep?" National Sleep Foundation, http://sleepfoundation.org/how-sleep-works/what-happens-when-you-sleep.

6.   Schocker, "Your Body Does Incredible Things."

7.   Elaine Magee, "Your 'Hunger Hormones,'" WebMD, http://www.webmd.com/diet/features/your-hunger-hormones.

8.   Helen Kollias, Leptin, Ghrelin, and Weight Loss," Precision Nutrition, http://www.precisionnutrition.com/leptin-ghrelin-weight-loss.

9.   Robert Portman, "Sleep Your Way Thin: 4 Benefits of Better Sleep," Pacific Health, http://www.pacifichealthlabs.com/blog/better-sleep/.

4.3: Get Moving

1. "Psychological Benefits of Exercise," Association for Applied Sport Psychology, http://www.appliedsportpsych.org/resource-center/health-fitness-resources/psychological-benefits-of-exercise/.

2. James Fell, "Exercise: Alternative Reward for Those Battling Addiction," *Chicago Tribune,* June 12, 2013, http://articles.chicagotribune.com/2013-06-12/health/sc-health -0612-fitness-fight -addiction-with-exerci-20130612_1_todd-crandell-drug-addiction -reward.

3. "Top 10 Reasons to Strength Train," Workouts Unlimited, www .workoutsunlimited.com/10-reasons-to-strength-train.html.

4. "Target Heart Rates," American Heart Association, June 8, 2015, http://www.heart.org/HEARTORG/GettingHealthy/PhysicalActivity/ FitnessBasics/Target-Heart-Rates_UCM_434341_Article.jsp.

5. Jennifer Wolfe, "What Is CrossFit?" How Stuff Works, http://health. howstuffworks.com/wellness/diet-fitness/exercise/what-is-crossfit.htm.

6. Michael Franco, "10 Health Benefits of Swimming," How Stuff Works, http://health.howstuffworks.com/wellness/aging/retirement/10-health -benefits-of-swimming.htm#page=1.

4.4: Eating Clean

1. Gabriel, *The Gabriel Method,* 12.

2. "Macronutrients: The Importance of Carbohydrate, Protein, and Fat," McKinley Health Center, http://www.mckinley.illinois.edu/handouts/ macronutrients.htm.

3. Sue Roberts, "What Are the Biggest Reasons Your Body Needs Protein?" SFGate, http://healthyeating.sfgate.com/biggest-reasons-body -needs-protein-5504.html.

4. Susan Reynolds, "The Skinny on Brain Fats," *Prime Your Gray Cells blog,* posted September 22, 2011, Psychology Today, https:// www.psychologytoday.com/blog/prime-your-gray-cells/201109/ the-skinny-brain-fats.

5. Joyce Hendley, "Q. Can Coconut Oil Help You Lose Weight?" EatingWell, January/February 2009, http://www.eatingwell .com/nutrition_health/nutrition _news_information/can_coconut _oil_help_you_lose_weight%20.

6.   "The Truth About Your Food with Food, Inc. Filmmaker Rober Kenner," YouTube, July 17, 2012, https://www.youtube.com/watch?v=2Oq24hITFTY. http://www.monsanto.com/food-inc/pages/default.aspx.

7.   "Dirty Dozen" and "Clean Fifteen," Environmental Working Group, http://www.ewg.org/foodnews/index.php.

8.   "What is GMO?" Non-GMO Project, http://www.nongmoproject.org/learn-more/what-is-gmo/.

9.   "GMOs in Our Food System," Just Food, http://justfood.org/farm-to-pantry/gmos-our-food-system.

10. "GMO Facts," Non-GMO Project, http://www.nongmoproject.org/learn-more/.

11. S. Ahmed, K. Guillem, Y. Vandaele, "Sugar Addiction: Pushing the Drug-Sugar Analogy to the Limit," *Current Opinion in Clinical Nutrition and Metabolic Care,* 16, 4, (2013): 434-439. http://www.ncbi.nlm.nih.gov/pubmed/23719144.

12. "Glycemic Index for Sweeteners," Sugar-Sweetener-Guide, http://www.sugar-and-sweetener-guide.com/glycemic-index-for-sweeteners.html.

13. Hethir Rodriguez, "Does Stevia Cause Infertility?" The Natural Fertility Company, http://natural-fertility-info.com/does-stevia-cause-infertility.html; Jacob Teitelbaum, "Effective Natural Treatment for Infertility," Stevia.com, http://www.stevia.com/Stevia_Article.aspx?Id=2432.

14. Lauren Geertsen, "Why I Quit Stevia," Empowered Sustenance, June 5, 2013, http://empoweredsustenance.com/is-stevia-bad-for-you/.

15. Joseph Mercola, "'Sweet' Isn't All There Is to Aspartame and Other Artificial Sweeteners," Mercola.com, http://www.mercola.com/Downloads/bonus/aspartame/report.aspx.

16. Joseph Mercola, "New Study of Splenda (Sucralose) Reveals Shocking Information About Potential Harmful Effects," Mercola.com, February 10, 2009, http://articles.mercola.com/sites/articles/archive/2009/02/10/new-study-of-splenda-reveals-shocking-information-about-potential-harmful-effects.aspx.

17. "Superfoods You Need Now," Health.com, http://www.health.com/health/gallery/0,,20306775,00.html.

18. "Chia Seed," Bob's Red Mill Natural Foods, http://www.bobsredmill .com/chia-seed.html.

19. Kris Gunnars, "11 Proven Health Benefits of Chia Seeds," Authority Nutrition, http://authoritynutrition.com/11-proven-health-benefits -of-chia-seeds/.

20. "The Health Benefits of Goji Berries," The Healthy Eating Site, http:// thehealthyeatingsite.com/the-health-benefits-of-goji-berries/.

21. Derek Bryan, "What are the Health Benefits of Dried Goji Berries?" LiveStrong.com, April 21, 2015, http://www.livestrong.com/article/ 341738-what-are-the-health -benefits-of-dried-goji-berries/.

22. "Hemp Seeds," Pure Healing Foods, http://www.purehealingfoods .com/hempHeartsInfo.php.

23. Laura Dolson, "Flax Seed: The Low Carb Whole Grain," About.com, June 29, 2015, http://lowcarbdiets.about.com/od/whattoeat/a/flaxinfo .htm.

24. Katherine Tweed, "The Truth About Kale," WebMD, June 19, 2014, http://www.webmd.com/food-recipes/kale-nutrition-and-cooking.

25. Karen Ansel, "Is Gluten Bad for You?" Women's Health, November 6, 2010, http://www.womenshealthmag.com/health/gluten-free-diet.

26. "What is Celiac Disease?" Celiac Disease Foundation, http://celiac.org/ celiac-disease/what-is-celiac-disease/.

27. Steve Kamb, "The Beginner's Guide to the Paleo Diet," Nerd Fitness, October 4, 2010, http://www.nerdfitness.com/blog/2010/10/04/the -beginners-guide -to-the-paleo-diet/.

28. "Gut and Psychology Syndrome," GAPSdiet, http://www.shop.gapsdiet .com/product.sc?productId=1&categoryId=7.

29. Christian Nordqvist, "What is the Mediterranean Diet?" Medical News Today, May 28, 2015 http://www.medicalnewstoday.com/ articles/149090.php.

30. The website of Dr. Peter J. D'Adamo & The Blood Type Diet, http:// www.dadamo.com, is a good source for further information on this method.

4.5: Detoxing for a Better Life

1. "About Air Toxics," U.S. Environmental Protection Agency, June 21, 2012, http://www.epa.gov/oar/toxicair/newtoxics.html.

2. Donna Gates, "The Most Common Sources of Toxins Trapped in Your Body and the Most Efficient Way to Eliminate Them," Body Ecology, http://bodyecology.com/articles/most_common_sources_of_toxins.php#.VG41Qr74vGw.

3. Mark Hyman, "How Toxins Make You Fat: 4 Steps to Get Rid of Toxic Weight," Dr. Mark Hyman, October 18, 2014, http://drhyman.com/blog/2012/02/20/how-toxins-make-you-fat-4-steps-to-get-rid-of-toxic-weight/.

4. Lipman, Frank, "What Do You Mean by Detox?" Dr. Frank Lipman, http://www.drfranklipman.com/what-do-you-mean-by-detox/.

5. Adam Hadhazy, "Think Twice: How the Gut's 'Second Brain' Influences Mood and Well-Being," Scientific American, February 12, 2010, http://www.scientificamerican.com/article/gut-second-brain/.

6. Glenn Ellis, "Strategies for Well-Being: Bowel Movements: Sinkers or Floaters?" Electronic Urban Report, March 10, 2011, http://www.eurweb.com/2011/03/strategies-for-well-being-bowel-movements-sinkers-or-floaters/.

7. Mayo Clinic Staff, "Dietary Fiber: Essential for a Healthy Diet," Mayo Clinic, http://www.mayoclinic.org/healthy-living/nutrition-and-healthy-eating/in-depth/fiber/art-20043983.

8. Recommended websites for doing a long-term cleanse: The Juice Lady, http://www.juiceladycherie.com/Juice/; Standard Process, http://www.standardprocess.com/Standard-Process/Purification-Program#.VFkKL0R9lec; Baseline Nutritionals, https://www.baselinenutritionals.com/shop.php.

9. "1-2-3 Start Your Juice Feasting Cleanse!" Raw Juice Guru, http://rawjuiceguru.com/juice-feasting-2/.

10. "Water Fasting," All About Fasting, http://www.allaboutfasting.com/water-fasting.html.

11. Daniel 1:12–15, ESV.

4.6: Nutritional Supplements

1. "Inflammation (Chronic)," Life Extension, http://www.lef.org/protocols/health-concerns/chronic-inflammation/page-01.

2. eicosapentaenoic acid (EPA) and docosahexaenoic acid (DHA).

3. α-linolenic acid (ALA).

4. "Vitamin D," U.S. Department of Health & Human Services, November 10, 2014, http://ods.od.nih.gov/factsheets/VitaminD -HealthProfessional/.

5. Bo Wagner, "21 Benefits of Enzymes and Why You Need Them," Generation Rescue, May 18, 2012, http://www.generationrescue.org/ latest-news/nutrition/21-benefits -of-enzymes-and-why-you-need-them/.

6. "Food Without Enzymes?" European Food Information Council, June 2006, http://www.eufic.org/article/en/expid/review-food-without -enzymes/.

7. "Digestion Problems & the Immune System," Benjamin Associates, http://immunedisorders.homestead.com/digestion.html.

8. "10 Benefits of Turmeric," Top 10 Remedies, http://www .top10homeremedies.com/kitchen-ingredients/10-health-benefits-of -turmeric.html/3.

9. Elizabeth Renter, "How to Optimize Turmeric Absorption for Super-Boosted Benefits," Natural Society, September 17, 2013, http:// naturalsociety.com/turmeric-absorption-super-benefits-black -pepper/.

10. "Apple Cider Vinegar for Health and Well Being," Earth Clinic, May 4, 2015, http://www.earthclinic.com/remedies/acvinegar.html.

11. "Organic India Turmeric, 90-Count," Amazon, http://www.amazon .com/dp/B000YC70XY/ref=sr_ph?ie=UTF8&qid=1417654931&sr =1&keywords=organic+turmeric.

12. Earth Clinic, "Apple Cider Vinegar."

13. Kris Gunnars, "6 Proven Benefits of Apple Cider Vinegar," Authority Nutrition, http://authoritynutrition.com/6-proven-health-benefits -of-apple-cider-vinegar/.

14. Katie, "Oil Pulling for Oral Health, Wellness Mama, http:// wellnessmama.com/7866/oil-pulling-for-oral-health/.

15. "Natural Calm," Natural Vitality, "Natural Calm," Natural Vitality, http://naturalvitality.com/natural-calm/.

16. Edward Group, "10 Amazing Benefits of Chlorophyll," Global Healing Center, January 6, 2014, http://www.globalhealingcenter.com/ natural-health/10-amazing-benefits-of-chlorophyll/.

17. "Melatonin and Sleep," National Sleep Foundation, http:// sleepfoundation.org/sleep-topics/melatonin-and-sleep.

18. Michele Vieux, "Top 7 Supplements for Athletes," CrossFit Invictus, http://www.crossfitinvictus.com/blog/top-7-supplements-for-athletes/.

19. Jennifer Nall, "What Does Glutamine Do for Your Muscles?" Livestrong.com, January 15, 2014, http://www.livestrong.com/article/440157-what-does-glutamine-do-for-your-muscles/.

20. David Galanis, "The Benefits of Glutamine," Bodybuilding.com, March 17, 2015, http://www.bodybuilding.com/fun/glutamine.htm.

21. "Quercetin," WebMD, http://www.webmd.com/vitamins-supplements/ingredientmono-294-quercetin.aspx?activeingredientid =294&activeingredientname=quercetin.

Chapter 5: Adrenal and Thyroid Health

1. Lyle H. Miller and Alma D. Smith, "Stress: The Different Kinds of Stress," American Psychological Association, http://www.apa.org/helpcenter/stress-kinds.aspx.

2. "Stress Effects," The American Institute of Stress, http://www.stress .org/stress-effects/.

3. Yagana Shah, "New Study Proves that Laughter Really is the Best Medicine," Huffington Post, April 22, 2014, http://www .huffingtonpost.com/2014/04/22/laughter-and-memory _n_5192086 .html.

4. "The Invisible Clock-II," Time Now, Inc., http://www.invisibleclock .com.

5. "Licorice Root (Glycyrrhiza Glabra)," Herbwisdom.com, http://www .herbwisdom.com/herb-licorice-root.html.

6. "General Information/Press Room," American Thyroid Association, http://www.thyroid.org/media-main/about-hypothyroidism/

7. Suzy Cohen, *Thyroid Healthy* (n.p.: Dear Pharmacist Incorporated, 2014), 20.

8. "Protein Fact Sheet," The Dr. Oz Show, May 16, 2013, http://www .doctoroz.com/article/protein-fact-sheet.

9. Go to the website of Standard Process: https://www.standardprocess .com/Home.

Chapter 6: Essential Oils

1. David Stewart, *The Healing Oils of the Bible* (Marble Hill, Mo.: CARE Publications, 2003), 101.

2. Ibid., 55.

3. *Essential Oils Desk Reference* (Orem, Utah: Life Science Publishing, 2014), 1.23.

4. Ibid.

5. Christa Black Gifford, "Do Essential Oils Really Work?" Christa Black, September 14, 2014, http://christablack.com/2014/09/do-essential-oils-really-work/.

6. "Reflexology Foot Chart - sole," how-to-do-Reflexology.com, http://www.how-to-do-reflexology.com/reflexologyfootmap.html.

7. Debbie McFarland, *Inspired by Essential Oils: Basic Guide* (lulu.com 2013), 98.

8. http://essentialoilbenefits.com/best-essential-oils-for-the-treatment-of-hemorrhoids/.

9. http://janasapothecary.com.

10. "Essential Oil Blend for Supporting Healthy Thyroid Levels," Green Living Ladies, February 6, 2014, www.greenlivingladies.com/2014/02/essential-oil-blend-for-hypothyroidism.html.

11. www.facebook.com/livelaughloveoils.

Chapter 7: The Skinny Obsession

1. "11 Facts About Eating Disorders," DoSomething.org, https://www.dosomething.org/facts/11-facts-about-eating-disorders.

2. Psalm 18:24, MSG.

Chapter 8: Spirit Health

1. Mark 8:22-26.

2. "What is 'Rhema'?" Advanced Training Institute International, http://ati.iblp.org/ati/family/articles/concepts/rhema/.

Recipes

1. Herzog, Natural to Supernatural Health , 72.

About Beni Johnson

BENI JOHNSON is an author, pastor and conference speaker. Together, she and her husband, Bill Johnson, are the Senior Pastors at Bethel Church in Redding, California. Beni is a mother to three children, along with their spouses and the grandmother to 9 grandchildren. Beni has traveled all over the world speaking at various churches bringing a message of peace, intercession and now, health. As she traveled, she noticed a growing number of individuals who were not educated on how to properly maintain their health. This, along with her compassion for people, has caused her to actively pursue bringing awareness regarding health. She is passionate in seeing and helping people reach their healthiest potential as they realize that they are destined for greatness in every part of their lives.

You can find Beni on instagram at @grandmaswithmuscles and Facebook at www.facebook.com/Grandmaswithmuscles or on her blog www.grandmaswithmuscles.com

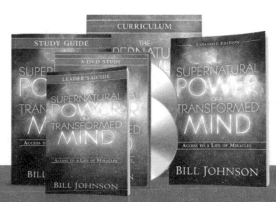

YOUR HEALTHY & FREE LIFESTYLE IS JUST ONE DECISION AWAY...

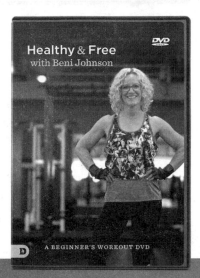

EXCERCISE.

In this workout DVD, Beni Johnson gives you fun, easy-to-follow exercises that leave you without excuse.

She makes working out so easy and fun that no matter how busy your schedule is, you can still make one of the most important investments of all: a healthy lifestyle!

Beni gives you over two hours of exciting and enjoyable workouts that will show you...

- How to exercise anywhere... from the comfort of your own home to the scenic environment of a park
- How to comfortably and effectively use equipment in your home
- How to confidently use gym machines to maximize your workout impact and effectiveness

Once you begin the journey and start feeling the results in your body, you will make working out a regular part of your schedule that will set you on course for a lifetime of living healthy and free!

Looking for more from
BENI JOHNSON AND BETHEL CHURCH?

Purchase additional resources—CDs, DVDs, digital
downloads, music—from Beni Johnson and the
Bethel team at the **online Bethel store.**

Visit www.bjm.org for more information on
Bill Johnson, to view his speaking itinerary, or to
look into additional teaching resources.

To order Bethel Church resources,
visit http://store.ibethel.org

Subscribe to Bethel.TV to access the latest sermons,
worship sets, and conferences from Bethel Church.
To subscribe, visit www.bethel.tv

Become part of a Supernatural Culture that is
transforming the world and *apply* for the
Bethel School of Supernatural Ministry

For more information, visit bssm.net

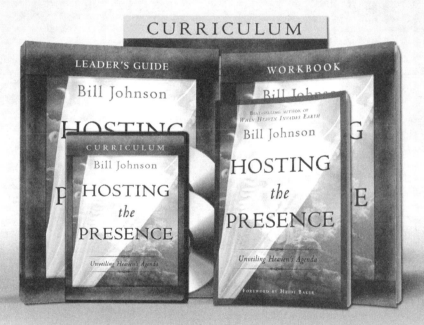
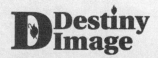

Healthy & Free

A JOURNEY TO WELLNESS FOR YOUR BODY, SOUL, AND SPIRIT

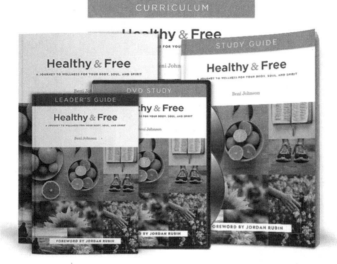

Experience Heaven's Health!

Beni Johnson received a life-changing revelation about how anyone can start walking in holistic health—including you! Jesus died for your spirit, soul, and body. This means you can experience His resurrection life in all three areas!

Christians should be the healthiest people on earth because they understand God has made their bodies His temple. Unfortunately, many people focus on one area of health while neglecting the others. This can lead to spiritual disconnection, bad eating habits, depression, poor rest, and lack of exercise.

In the *Healthy and Free* video curriculum, Beni personally teaches you how to:

- **Find your why:** Learn the motivating secret to pursuing a healthy lifestyle as your new normal.
- **Unlock the connection:** Discover the many ways your spirit, soul, and body are interconnected and how health in one area directly affects another.
- **Start simple:** Receive practical and easy-to-implement steps to begin walking in health right now.

The Great Physician desires you to walk in Heaven's health. Get aligned with God's divine design today and experience freedom—body, soul, and spirit!

INCLUDED IN THIS CURRICULUM:

8-Session DVD Study • Leader's Guide • Study Guide • *Healthy and Free* Book

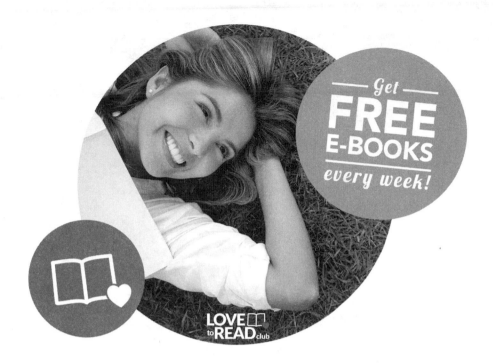

Get — FREE E-BOOKS every week!

LOVE to READ club

JOIN *the* CLUB

As a member of the **Love to Read Club,** receive exclusive offers for FREE, 99¢ and $1.99 e-books* every week. Plus, get the **latest news** about upcoming releases from **top authors** like these...

DESTINYIMAGE.COM/FREEBOOKS

| T.D. JAKES | BILL JOHNSON | CINDY TRIMM | JIM STOVALL | BENI JOHNSON | MYLES MUNROE |

LOVE to READ club